BIOCHEMISTRY RESEARCH TRENDS

CAROTENOIDS

BIOSYNTHESIS, PROPERTIES AND PHYSIOLOGICAL EFFECTS

Biochemistry Research Trends

Additional books in this series can be found on Nova's website under the Series tab.

Additional e-books in this series can be found on Nova's website under the eBooks tab.

BIOCHEMISTRY RESEARCH TRENDS

CAROTENOIDS

BIOSYNTHESIS, PROPERTIES AND PHYSIOLOGICAL EFFECTS

HANNE LEIF
AND
FELIX ULRIK
EDITORS

nova
science publishers
New York

NOTICE TO THE READER

Library of Congress Cataloging-in-Publication Data

ISBN: 978-1-53612-685-3

Published by Nova Science Publishers, Inc. † New York

CONTENTS

PREFACE

In the first chapter, Saraid Mora Rochín, PhD, Jorge Milán Carrillo, PhD, and Cuauhtémoc Reyes Moreno, PhD review the function of food carotenoids in oxidative stress-induced human disease prevention. In the second chapter, Andrêssa S. Fernandes, Pricila N. Pinheiro, Mariany C. Deprá, Eduardo Jacob-Lopes, and Leila Q. Zepka discuss the biosynthesis of carotenoids and bioactive caortenoids from microalgae, as well as their applications. Alexis Marsol-Vall, Albert Tomàs, Mercè Balcells, Francisca Vilaró, and Ramon Canela-Garayoa present a study where cuticles of four apple varieties were studied for their carotenoid content in the third chapter. In the fourth chapter, Joanna Igielska-Kalwat reviews the cosmetic applications of carotenoids, including their antiaging properties.

Chapter 1 - Normal human metabolism produces free radicals, and the over production of these biomolecules leads to increased oxidative stress and contributes to the development of chronic diseases. Recent studies have shown that secondary plant metabolites contain bioactive compounds with functional properties and beneficial effects for human health. The consumption of fruits, vegetables, and grains (wheat and maize) has increased due to their bioactive composition and antioxidant potential, which could mitigate the damage and negative effects of the oxidative stress process. Carotenoids are considered nutraceuticals for their functional properties and their role as antioxidants, acting as physical quenchers of singlet oxygen, and scavengers of other reactive oxygen species. Carotenoids are considered the most important group of pigments with approximately 750 moieties known. Carotenoids such as lutein, zeaxanthin, β-cryptoxanthin, carotenes, and their metabolites play a protective role in reactive oxygen species-mediated disorders such as: cardiovascular disease, some types of cancer, and neurological, as well as photosensitive and eye-related disorders. While fruits and vegetables constitute the main source of carotenoids in human diet, recent studies have shown that grains like maize are a functional source of carotenoids, mainly of lutein and zeaxanthin. This chapter is focused on the role of food carotenoids in the prevention of oxidative stress-induced human diseases.

Chapter 2 - The carotenoids are isoprenoids, highly unsatured, lipophilic, featuring a variety cores from yellow to red. Appoximately 750 naturally occurring, and many of this tetraterpenes are produced from microalgae. The composition of carotenoids from microalgae can still be complex, with structural characteristics very different from those commonly found in foods, such as a greater number of carbon atoms, of c.d.b., and of hydroxyl groups, which all contribute to their great antioxidant capacity. These compounds have properties that result in biological functions beneficial to human health, such as cellular protection against free radicals, it is know that the antioxidant properties of the carotenoids are are closely related to their chemical structure. Carotenoids are a source of several bioactive compounds with great otential for applications in food, cosmect, and pharmaceutical industries. Thus, the chapter is organized in three major topics. (1) fundamental aspects of structure and biosynthesis of carotenoids from microalgae, (2) bioactive carotenoids from microalgae, (3) examples of novelty to industrial applications.

Chapter 3 - A statical approach based on Principal Component Analysis (PCA) was performed to study the contents of carotenoids present in the cuticle of four apple varieties (Golden Reinders; Fuji Zhen Aztec; Fuji Fubrax and Superchief) with different scald susceptibility after harvest and low temperature storage. The scald phenomenon results from the damage and death within the surface layers of cells in localized regions of apple and pears. The authors' study demonstrates that the four apples varieties showed different carotenoid profiles in the cuticle and also that the fate of these carotenoids was different during the conservation of the four varieties at low temperature for 7 month. The two PCs explained 81.4% of the variability at harvest. A clear separation in PC1 between the two Fuji cultivars and Golden Reinders and Superchief was observed. In addition, the loadings plot indicated that Fuji cultivars had a more heterogeneous content of carotenoids, while Superchief and Golden Reinders were highly correlated with β-carotene, (all-*E*)-lutein and (all-*E*)-violaxanthin. In contrast, more biosynthetic evolved oxidized carotenoids, such as luteoxanthin isomers, neochrome and neoxhanthin isomers, would explain the behaviour of the Fuji varieties. After seven months of cold storage PC1 and PC2 explained 86.4% of the variability of carotenoid. A clear separation of the four cultivars was observed. In this regard, as in samples at harvest, the scores plot revealed separation between Fuji cultivars and Golden Reinders, and Superchief in the PC1. However, in this case, a separation between Golden Reinders and Superchief is shown in PC2. The loadings plot indicates that Fuji cultivars presented a higher correlation with diverse carotenoids, mainly those same oxocarotenoids as at the time of harvesting. Superchief was still positively correlated with the content of (all-*E*)-lutein. (9'Z)-Neoxanthin also appeared to be responsible for the PC1 differentiation between Golden Reinders and Superchief, and the two Fuji varieties. In addition, neochrome and auroxanthin B, and β-carotene would participate in the PC2 differentiation between Golden Reinders and Superchief. The authors hypothesize that the different scald susceptibility of the four apples varieties could partially be a consequence of these differences in profile and fate. Indeed, carotenoids are considered natural antioxidants, however their antioxidant capability depends on their chemical structure.

Chapter 4 - According to recent canons of beauty, the skin touched by the sun signifies healthy lifestyle and wellbeing. The skin makes an excellent model to study the process of ageing. It is directly exposed to destructive effect of the elements and hence more prone to ageing than other organs of the body. Ageing is a multifactorial process controlled by both genetic and environmental factors. Carotenoids, which belong to the best known natural antioxidants, have been for many years the subject of studies aimed at their possible application in cosmetic industry. Carotenoids contain 11 coupled double bonds, so they can be classified as polyisoprenoids and they are weakly polar. Provitamin A assists in regeneration of tissues, prevents degeneration of epithelium lining the alimentary tract mucosa, lacrimal glands and salivary glands as well as urinary tracts.

In: Carotenoids
Editors: Hanne Leif and Felix Ulrik
ISBN: 978-1-53612-685-3

Chapter 1

Carotenoids as Functional Ingredients

Jorge Milán Carrillo, PhD[1], Saraid Mora Rochín, PhD[1,*] and Cuauhtémoc Reyes Moreno, PhD[1],
[1]Facultad de Ciencias Químico Biológicas,
Universidad Autónoma de Sinaloa,
Culiacán Sinaloa, México

Abstract

Normal human metabolism produces free radicals, and the over production of these biomolecules leads to increased oxidative stress and contributes to the development of chronic diseases. Recent studies have shown that secondary plant metabolites contain bioactive compounds with functional properties and beneficial effects for human health. The consumption of fruits, vegetables, and grains (wheat and maize) has increased due to their bioactive composition and antioxidant potential, which could mitigate the damage and negative effects of the oxidative stress process. Carotenoids are considered nutraceuticals for their functional properties and their role as antioxidants, acting as physical quenchers of singlet oxygen, and scavengers of other reactive oxygen species. Carotenoids are considered the most important group of pigments with approximately 750 moieties known. Carotenoids such as lutein,

[*]Corresponding Author: Blvd. de las Américas y Josefa Ortiz de Domínguez, Ciudad Universitaria, Facultad de Ciencias Químico Biológicas, Culiacán Sinaloa México. Email: smora@uas.edu.mx.

zeaxanthin, β-cryptoxanthin, carotenes, and their metabolites play a protective role in reactive oxygen species-mediated disorders such as: cardiovascular disease, some types of cancer, and neurological, as well as photosensitive and eye-related disorders. While fruits and vegetables constitute the main source of carotenoids in human diet, recent studies have shown that grains like maize are a functional source of carotenoids, mainly of lutein and zeaxanthin. This chapter is focused on the role of food carotenoids in the prevention of oxidative stress-induced human diseases.

Keywords: carotenoids, antioxidants, chronic diseases, functional ingredients

INTRODUCTION

Reactive oxygen species (ROS) and reactive nitrogen species (RNS) are generated by different cellular and metabolic sources, exposure to different physiochemical conditions or pathological states, and their accumulation in the human system is widely considered to cause chronic diseases (Valko et al. 2006; Rao and Rao 2007). ROS and RNS are well recognized for playing a dual role, both deleterious and beneficial on living systems (Valko et al. 2007). The most common ROS include: hydroxil, peroxide anion, and superoxide anion radicals. Under normal physiological conditions superoxide anion and the nitric oxide system are the main radicals generated by cells. These free radicals can alter proteins, lipids, and DNA triggering a number of human diseases (Finkel and Holbrook 2000; Rao and Rao 2007). Hence, the use of antioxidants can help the body tolerate the oxidative stress-induced damage (Dasgupta and Klein 2014; Baiano and Del Nobile 2016).

It has been demonstrated that plants contain secondary metabolites responsible for their bright colors. These bioactive compounds are phytochemicals known to possess antioxidant capacity and functional properties that are physiologically important for protecting human health. Animals and humans are unable to synthesize carotenoids de *novo*, therefore they must include them in a healthy diet (Stahl and Sies 2005; Eldahshan and Singab 2013; Alfieri et al. 2014).

The most abundant types of antioxidants in fruits, vegetables, and grains include: vitamin C, phenolic compounds and carotenoids, whereas tocotrienols and tocopherols are present in lower concentrations compared with grains (Kalt 2005). Epidemiological studies have shown that antioxidant compounds such as vitamin E and carotenoids (β-carotene, α-carotene, β-cryptoxanthin, lycopene, lutein, and zeaxanthin) contribute to prevent degenerative disorders, such as cardiovascular disease (CVD), diabetes, and several types of cancer (Rodriguez-Amaya and Kimura 2004; Maughan 2005; Singh and Goyal 2008; Gul et al. 2015).

The carotenoids comprise approximately 750 structurally different compounds of phytonutrients and 50 of them are present in a typical human diet. More than 20 carotenoids have been identified in human blood and tissues (prostate, eye macula and liver) (Jain et al. 1999; Khachik 2006; Prabhashankar-Arathi et al. 2015). Carotenoids are considered of great importance for their biological functions and are among the most abundant families of pigments in nature. They give fruits, vegetables, and grains their distinctive yellow, orange, and red color (Ndolo and Beta 2013; Corrales-Bañuelos et al. 2016). Carotenoids are important not only for coloring food, but as dietary sources of vitamins, and for their reported association with the reduction rates of coronary heart disease and some varieties of cancer (Figure 1). The first correlation between a high intake of carotenoids and health benefits appeared in the literature in the 1970's (Fraser and Bramley 2004). Thus far, the antioxidant and functional properties of carotenoids have been a major focus of research (Rao and Rao 2007; Gul et al. 2015; Corrales-Bañuelos et al. 2016).

Considering a nutritional approach, carotenoids are considered to be important bioactive compounds, and dietary ingestion as the only source to meet their requirements in humans and animals (Prabhashankar-Arathi et al. 2015). Recent studies indicate that fruits and vegetables are an important source of carotenoids in the human diet (Sommerburg et al. 1998; Rao and Rao 2007; Fiedor and Burda 2014). However, some grains may contain higher, while others lower content of carotenoids compared to fruits and vegetables (Abdel-Aal et al. 2002; Ndolo and Beta 2013). Although grains contain other bioactive compounds that complement those found in fruits and vegetables (Liu 2007).

Cereals such as maize have a complex matrix rich in bioactive compounds such as carotenoids, phenolics, and minerals, all of which have been reported to have antioxidant properties and to be associated with the prevention of chronic diseases (Hänsch and Mendel 2009; Da Silva-Messias et al. 2015). To date, there is a world-wide interest in functional foods. However, more information is needed regarding the levels of carotenoids that have health enhancing properties in fruits, vegetables and grain cereals. The purpose of this review is to discuss the literature focused on the functional properties and the beneficial effects of carotenoids in human health.

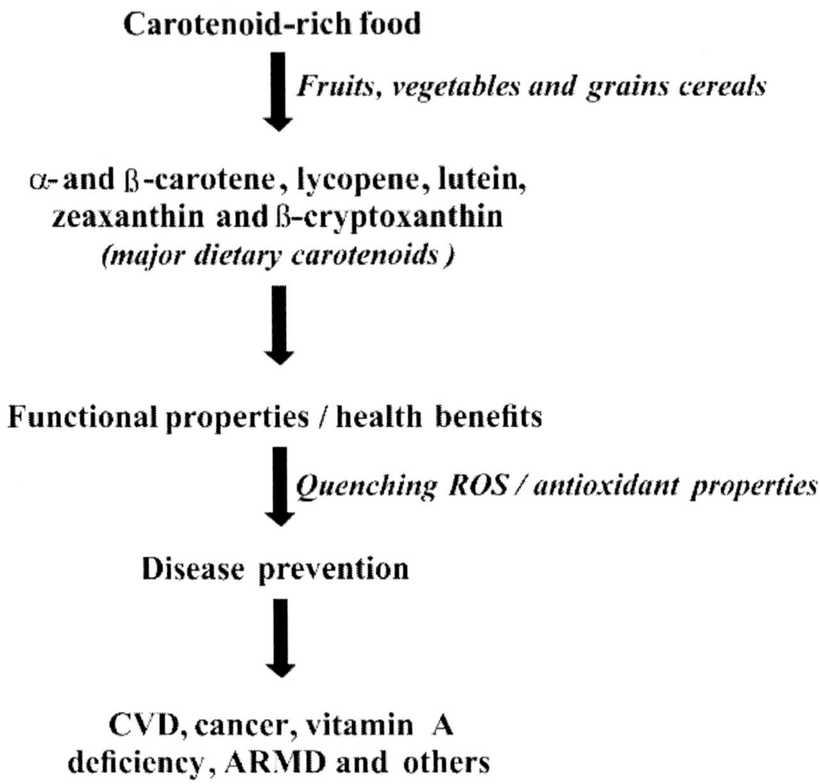

Figure 1. Functional properties of food carotenoids.

Chemical Properties of Carotenoids

Carotenoids are a family of pigmented compounds synthesized by plants and microorganisms (bacteria, yeast, and fungi). However, humans and animals cannot synthesize them (Rao and Rao 2007; Britton et al. 2009). In plants, carotenoids contribute to the photosynthetic machinery and protect them against photo-damage (Rao and Rao 2007; Fiedor and Burda 2014), while in animals, such as insects, fish, crustaceans and birds, carotenoids are responsible for their characteristic color (Stahl and Sies 2005). Carotenoids are intracellular compounds usually synthesized in membranes of mitochondria, chloroplasts, or endoplasmic reticulum (Margalith 1999). Carotenoids are highly hydrophobic and tend to be associated with lipids (oil, fat) or in hydrophobic structures such as membranes (Britton et al. 2008). Carotenoids of fruits, vegetables, and animal products are usually fat-soluble and are associated with lipid fractions, lipid portions of human tissues, cells (El-Qudah 2008), and the lipid core of the bilayer membrane (Britton et al. 2008). The orientation of a particular carotenoid in the membrane and its effect on membrane properties depends on its structural features such as the size and shape of the carotenoid, and the presence of functional groups (Britton et al. 2008).

Carotenoids are tetrapernoids composed by 40 carbon atoms built from four terpene units, each of these containing 10 carbon atoms. Their main chemical functions are determined by the extended system of conjugated double bonds, which is also responsible for their color (Britton 1995). They are categorized into two major groups: 1) those containing oxygen, known as xanthophylls (e.g., lutein, zeaxanthin, α-and β-cryptoxanthin), and 2) those that contain only hydrocarbons and do not contain oxygen, known as carotenes (e.g., α- and β-carotene, and lycopene) (Baiano and Del Nobile 2016) (Figure 2). Therefore, depending on the number of double bonds, a certain array of *cis*/*trans* (E/Z) configurations is possible for a given carotenoid (Britton et al. 1995).

The all-*trans* configurations are ubiquitously present, while several *cis* isomers of carotenoids are present in blood and tissues such as prostate, breast, adrenal glands, and liver (Jain et al. 1999; Melendez-Martinez et al. 2004; Yahia and Ornelas 2010). However, when fruits and vegetables are processed, it results in an increase from 10 to 39% in *cis*-isomers. The all-*trans* structure is thermodynamically most stable (Yahia and Ornelas-Paz 2010). Nonetheless, the degree of isomerisation is directly correlated with the intensity and duration of the heating process (Eldahshan and Singab 2013). It has been observed that high temperatures and short times are preferred conditions for processing carotenoid-containing foods, yet extreme heat can result in oxidative destruction of carotenoids (Agarwal and Rao 2000; Delgado-Vargas and Paredes-López 2003). Other factors that can influence the stability and nutritional value of matrix foods include temperature, light, and pH (Melendez-Martinez et al. 2004). However, it is important to keep in mind, that food processing and heat treatment cause the mechanical breakdown of the tissue, releasing the carotenoids and improving their absorption (Gärtner et al. 1997). The type of food matrix in which carotenoids are located is a major factor influencing their bioavailability (Haskell 2012; Gul et al. 2015).

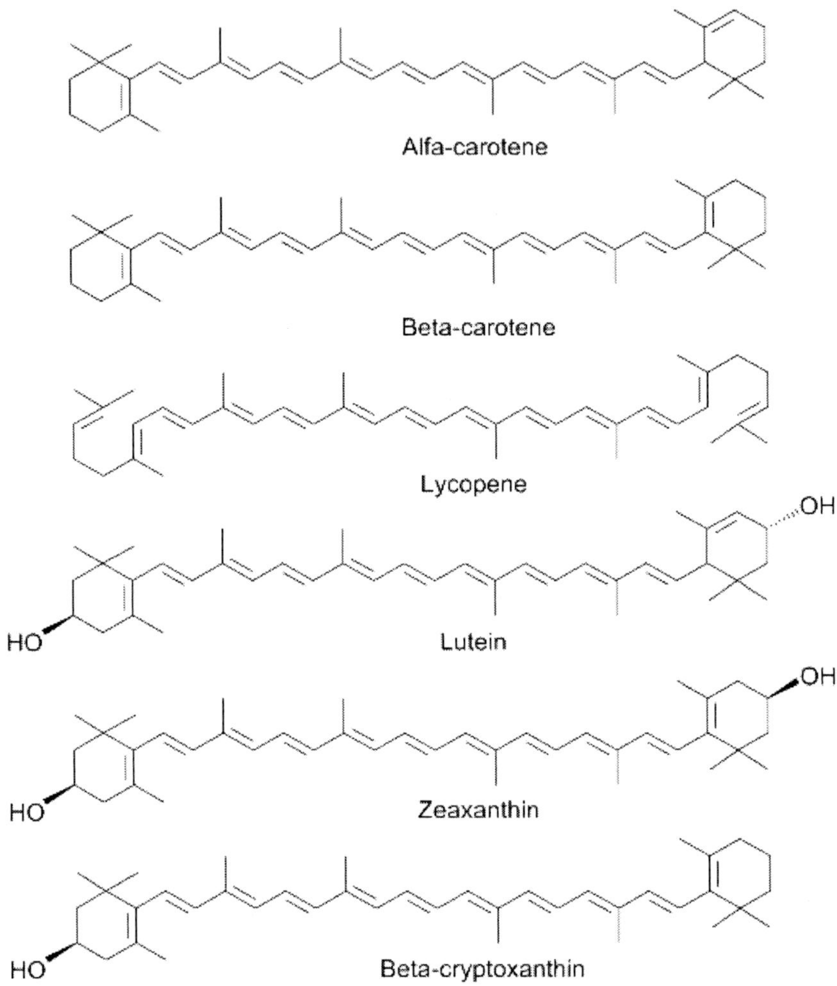

Figure 2. Chemical structure of major dietary carotenoids.

The relatively low bioavailability of carotenoids from natural sources has been attributed to the fact that they exist either as crystals or are located within protein complexes that are not fully released in the gastrointestinal tract during digestion (Williams et al. 1998; Gul et al. 2015).

The mechanism of intestinal absorption of carotenoids occurs by passive diffusion after being incorporated into the micelles, which are formed by dietary fat and bile. They are then incorporated into lipoproteins and released into the blood stream (Olson 1994; Parker 1988; Rao and Rao 2007). It has been reported that only about 5% of the carotenoids are absorbed in the intestine, whereas >50% are absorbed from micellar solution (Olson 1994). Because there are numerous factors affecting the bioavailability, absorption, transport, metabolism, and storage of carotenoids (Fiedor and Burda 2014), the exact mechanism by which carotenes exert their actions *in vivo* are still far from being understood.

Functional Properties of Carotenoids

Antioxidant Capacity of Carotenoids

Reactive oxygen and nitrogen species are generated during aerobic metabolism and pathological processes, such species are highly reactive and can induce the irreversible oxidation of diverse biomolecules such as lipids, proteins, carbohydrates, and DNA (Valko et al. 2006; Dasgupta and Klein 2014). Lipids are the major targets for oxidative damage induced by free radicals. Lipid peroxidation generates cell membrane damage by altering the membrane fluidity and permeability (Aikens and Dix 1991; Dasgupta and Klein 2014). Oxidation of proteins by ROS and RNS involves side chains of all amino acid residues of proteins (Stadtman 2004). Likewise, hydroxyl radicals are known to damage DNA, leading to disorders in purine and pyrimidine bases and the deoxyribose backbone (Halliwell and Gutteridge 1999). DNA damage is implicated in mutagenesis, carcinogenesis, and aging. Oxidative stress can also damage mitochondrial DNA and lead to disorders associated with aging and cancer development in various tissues (Dasgupta and Klein 2014).

Carotenoids and other bioactive compounds provide protection against some types of cancer, coronary vascular disease (CDV), age-related macular degeneration (ARMD), and the risk of vitamin A deficiency (Jaswir et al. 2011; Yahia and Ornelas-Paz 2010).

The way carotenes exert their protective actions most likely involve the scavenging of two of the ROS: singlet molecular oxygen, and peroxyl radicals (Truscott 1990; Valko et al. 2007). They are also effective deactivators of electronically excited molecules involved in the generation of radicals and singlet oxygen (Truscott 1990; Young and Lowe 2001).

The antioxidant actions of carotenoids are based on their singlet oxygen quenching properties, and their ability to trap peroxyl radicals. The quenching activity of a carotenoid is mainly attributed to the number of conjugated double bonds of its structure while is influenced to a lesser extent by carotenoid groups (cyclic or acyclic), or the nature of substituents in carotenoids containing cyclic end groups (Krinsky 1998; Eldahshan and Singab 2013). Until now, it has been concluded that the number of conjugated double bonds is the most effective parameter for quenching properties because the activity of carotenoids increases as the number of the conjugated double bonds in the carotenoids increases. Furthermore, the bioactivity of carotenoids has been associated with their antioxidant capacity *in vivo* and *in vitro* (Delgado-Vargas and Paredes-López 2003; Tanaka et al. 2012). For instance, β-carotene treatment in human dermal fibroblasts (FEK4) exposed to UVA light was able to suppress the heme oxygenase-1 gene upregulation in a dose dependent manner (Elliott 2005). Likewise, in human liver cells (HepG2), carotenoids were able to decrease the oxidant-induced lipid peroxidation (Martin et al. 1996).

β-carotene is a promising potent antioxidant because of its ability as a singlet oxygen quencher. Such antioxidant capacity is due to the structure of conjugated double bonds and ionone rings, with capability of quenching up to 1,000 free radicals per molecule. Thus, it can prevent oxidative damage, alter transcriptional activity and prevent cellular damage (Abdel-Aal and Akhtar 2006; Singh and Goyal 2008; Qian et al. 2012; Gul et al. 2015). A study by Sindhu et al. (2010) reported lutein as a potent antioxidant *in vivo*. The authors gave oral lutein to mice for a month and observed an increase in the activity of the antioxidant defense enzymes: superoxide dismutase, catalase, glutatione reductase, and glutatione in blood and liver when compared to controls. Likewise, liver glutatione peroxidase and glutatione-S-transferase also increased their activity. On the other hand, it is important to note that high carotenoid concentrations may also induce a pro-oxidative effect, which could be modified by interactions with other nutrients (Eldahshan and Singab 2013).

Health Benefits of Carotenoids

Provitamin A Carotenoids and Prevention of Vitamin A Deficiency and Eye-Related Disorders

Carotenoids are divided in two classes: provitamin A and non-provitamin compounds. The contribution of provitamin A carotenoids to the daily vitamin A intake depends on dietary habits and available food sources. It has been estimated that carotenoids from fruits and vegetables provide more that 70% of the vitamin A intake in third world countries. However, intake must be corrected for bioequivalence, evaluating what portion of the ingested provitamin A carotenoids is absorbed, metabolized, and available as retinol or retinyl ester (Het-Hof et al. 2005; Stahl and Sies 2005).

Several studies have shown that the bioequivalence of plant-derived provitamin A carotenoids is much less than anticipated from studies using dietary supplements. As previously discussed, bioavailability and metabolism of carotenoids are affected by several factors including food matrix properties, preparation of the food, co-ingestion of fat and fiber, gastrointestinal tract diseases, vitamin A status, and malnutrition (Stahl and Sies 2005).

Provitamin A carotenoids such as α-, β-carotene, and β-cryptoxanthin, provide the primary dietary source of vitamin A. While α-carotene and β-cryptoxanthin produce one molecule of vitamin A, two molecules are generated from β-carotene. Hence, the consumption of provitamin A carotenoids can prevent vitamin A deficiency. Vitamin A deficiency is a serious global health problem that affects many people, especially children. In humans, this deficiency is associated with impaired iron mobilization, growth retardation, blindness, depressed immune response, increased susceptibility to infectious disease, and increased childhood mortality (Wurtzel et al. 2012). Carotenoids, particularly lutein and zeaxanthin, offer protection against eye diseases such as cataract and ARMD (Botella-Pavia and Rodríguez-Concepción 2006; Alfieri et al. 2014). Most likely, the mechanism of action of carotenoids for reducing the incidence of these diseases is quenching ROS (Fraser and Bramley 2004). Interestingly, it has been shown that the addition of lycopene to cell cultures prevents vacuolization in human lens epithelial cells (Mohanty et al. 2002). Likewise, other reports have shown the presence of lutein and zeaxanthin in the human macula, suggesting a role of these biocompounds in the macula protection from light-induced damage and scavenging of free radicals formed in the photoreceptors. However, it is still challenging to understand the presence of these specific carotenoids in the eye macula (Bone et al. 1997).

Carotenoids and Prevention of Coronary Vascular Disease

Carotenoids, as lipophilic compounds, are efficient scavengers of ROS within the hydrophobic parts of cell membranes and lipoproteins (Agarwal et al. 2012). ROS-mediated damage in atherosclerosis (hardening of the arteries) is the result of oxidative modification of low-density lipoproteins (LDL) in the arterial walls leading to coronary heart disease (Vogiatzi et al. 2009; Eldahshan and Singab 2013). This hypothesis is supported by observational and epidemiological studies that report that carotenoids, antioxidant vitamins, and the consumption of processed-tomato products can reduce LDL oxidation and oxidative stress at the site of the plaque formation (Mayne 1996; Hadley et al. 2003).

β-carotene supplementation (with or without aspirin) results in a significant reduction of vascular accidents in individuals with ischemic heart disease (Hennekens et al. 1996). However, clinical and intervention studies are contradictory. In some cases, it can be clearly observed a positive effect of β-carotene on cardiovascular disease, while in others, little or no correlation between them can be found, and sometimes an inverse relationship has been reported (Fiedor and Burda 2014).

Due to the abundance of CVD, studies on factors that prevent or delay its development are of special importance. The results of reports of the association of carotenoids (mainly β-carotene, α-carotene, lycopene, lutein, zeaxanthin and β-cryptoxanthin) with the risk of CVD and atherosclerosis have been summarized by Mayne (1996) and more recently by Voutilainen et al. (2006). These authors pointed out that there is a positive correlation between a high intake of carotenoid-rich fruits and vegetables and the reduction of CVD morbidity and mortality (Fiedor and Burda 2014). However, the biological mechanisms for such protection are currently unclear.

Carotenoids and Cancer Chemoprevention

Carotenoids by themselves or in combination with other bioactive compounds could protect from cancer risk due to their antimutagenic properties and their well-known ability to scavenge free radicals, delay tumor development, and improve the immune response (Tanaka et al. 2012).

Carotenoids have been extensively studied using *in vitro* experiments. These studies have shown that carotenoids can inhibit cell proliferation, transformation and micronucleus formation, and can modulate gene expression (Fraser and Bramley 2004). Likewise, epidemiological studies have demonstrated an association between a diet rich in β-carotene and the reduction of risk of cancer in stomach, lung, and other organs (Le-Marchand et al. 1993; van Poppel 1993; van Poppel and Goldbohom 1995; Eldahshan and Singab 2013). Similarly, *in vivo* studies have demonstrated that β-carotene can delay or prevent the induction of sarcomas and skin cancer in mice exposed to carcinogens (Smigel 1990; Eldahshan and Singab 2013).

Lycopene has been shown to be the main bioactive compound in tomatoes. Since 1995 Giovannuci and colleagues revealed an inverse relationship between the consumption of tomatoes and the risk of prostate cancer. Interestingly, in humans there is an increase in lycopene in serum and prostate when they consume tomatoes processed by heat treatment and oil vs.

when they consume raw tomatoes (Stahl and Sies 1992; Gärtner et al. 1997; Van Breeman et al. 2002; Giovannucci 2005). It has been also reported that tomato-based lycopene is more effective than lycopene supplementation (Agarwal and Rao 1998; Giovannucci 2005). Thus, suggesting that foods naturally rich in lycopene can be used in the prevention of prostate cancer. Besides prostate cancer, the protective effect of lycopene has been reported in other varieties of cancer including cervical, ovarian, breast, lung, gastrointestinal, and pancreatic cancer (Giovannucci 1999). Lycopene has also shown to decrease breast cancer risk. The mechanism of action of lycopene in the inhibition of breast cancer is associated with inhibition of cell cycle progression at the G_1 phase (Nahum et al. 2001). Similarly, *in vivo* studies have showed that β-carotene can delay or inhibit the development of sarcomas and skin cancer in mice exposed to carcinogens (Smigel 1990).

To date, α- and β-carotene, β-cryptoxanthin, lutein, and zeaxanthin are the major carotenoids with functional properties, and have been vigorously evaluated for their potential chemopreventive ability (Tanaka et al. 2012).

Conclusion

Carotenoids are important bioactive compounds known for their role as antioxidants and scavengers of free radicals. Carotenoids are found ubiquitously in fruits, vegetables, and grains, and to include these carotenoid-rich foods in a regular diet has been reported to be beneficial for human health. Evidence from epidemiological and clinical studies support a strong correlation with dietary intake of carotenoids and the reduction of vitamin A deficiency, age-related macular degeneration, certain types of cancer, and cardiovascular disease. Although, the antioxidant properties of some varieties of carotenoids have been reported *in vivo* and *in vitro*, these studies are mainly focused on provitamin A carotenoids. Thus, more studies that include non-provitamin compounds are necessary. In addition, future studies using dietary supplements should consider the stage of oxidative damage in order to establish the appropriate antioxidant supplementation. Only through such studies, our understanding of the role played by carotenoids and other bioactive compounds will be enhanced. Then, we would be able to develop complementary strategies for the prevention, treatment and management of human diseases.

References

Abdel-Aal, E. S. M. and Akhtar M. H. (2006). Recent advances in the analyses of carotenoids and their role in human health. *Current Pharmaceutical Analysis, 2,* 195-204.

Abdel-Aal, E. S. M., Young, J. C., Wood, P. J., Rabalski, I., Hucl, P., Falk D., Frégeau-Reid, J. (2002). Einkorn: A potential candidate for developing high lutein wheat. *Cereal Chemistry, 79*, 455-457.

Agarwal, M., Parameswari, R. P., Vasanthi, H. R., Das, D. K. (2012). Dynamic action of carotenoids in cardioprotection and maintenance of cardic health. *Molecules, 17*, 4755-4769.

Agarwal, S. and Rao, A. V. (2000). Carotenoids and chronic diseases. *Drug Metabolism and Drug Interaction, 17*, 189-210.

Agarwal, S. and Rao, A. V. (1998). Tomato lycopene and low density lipoprotein oxidation: a human dietary intervention study. *Lipids, 33*, 981-984.

Aikens, J. and Dix, T. A. (1991). Perhydroxyl radical (HOO•) initiated lipid-peroxidation-the role of fatty-acid hydroperoxides. *Journal Biological Chemistry, 266*, 15091-15098.

Alfieri, M., Hidalgo, A., Berardo, N., Redaelli, R. (2014). Carotenoid composition and heterotic effect in selected Italian maize germplasm. *Journal of Cereal Science, 59,* 181-188.

Baiano, A. and Del Nobile, M. A. (2016). Antioxidant compounds from vegetable matrices: Biosynthesis, occurrence, and extraction systems. *Critical Review in Food Science and Nutrition, 56,* 2053-2068.

Bone, R. A., Landrum, J. T., Friedes, L. M., Gomez, C. M., Kilburn, M. D., Menendez, E., Vidal, I., Wang, W. (1997). Distribution of lutein and zeaxanthin stereoisomers in the human retina. *Experimental Eye Research, 64*, 211-218.

Botella-Pavia, P. and Rodríguez-Concepción, M. (2006). Carotenoid biotechnology in plants for nutritionally improved foods. *Physiologia Plantarum, 126*, 369-381.

Britton G. (1995). Carotenes by their chemical structure. *American Journal of Nutrition*, *47*, 1990-2001.

Britton, G., Liaaen-Jensen, S., Pfander, H. (1995). *Carotenoids,* Vol. 1B*:* *Spectroscopy*, Basel, Switzerland: Birkhäuser Verlag.

Britton, G., Liaaen-Jensen, S., Pfander, H. (2009). Carotenoids. In: *Nutrition and health*, Vol. 5. Ch. 1. Basel, Switzerland: Birkhäuser Verlag.

Britton, G., Liaaen-Jensen, S., Pfender, H. (2008). *Special Molecules*: *Special properties*. *In*: *Carotenoids: Natural Functions,* Vol. 4 Ch. 1. Britton, G., Liaaen-Jensen, F., Pfander, H. (Eds.). Basel, Switzerland: Birkhäuser Verlag, pp. 1-6

Corrales-Bañuelos, A., Cuevas-Rodríguez, E. O., Gutiérrez-Uribe, J. A., Milán-Noris, E. M., Reyes-Moreno, C., Milán-Carrillo, J., Mora-Rochín, S. (2016). Carotenoid composition and antioxidant activity of tortillas elaborated from pigmented maize landrace by tradicional nixtamalization or lime cooking extrusion process. *Journal of Cereal Science, 69*, 64-70.

Dasgupta A. and Klein K. (2014). Antioxidants in food, vitamins and supplements: *Prevention and treatment of disease* (1rs ed.). San Diego, CA: Elsevier.

Da Silva-Messias, R., Galli, V., Delmar-Dos, S., Silva, A., Artigas-Schirmer, M., Valmor-Rombaldi, C. (2015). Micronutrient and Functional Compounds Biofortification of Maize Grains. *Critical Reviews in Food Science and Nutrition, 55*, 123-139.

Delgado-Vargas, F. and Paredes-López, O. (2003). *Natural Colorants for Food and Nutraceutical Uses* (1rs ed.). Boca Raton, FL: CRC PRESS.

Eldahshan, O. A. and Singab, A. N. B. (2013). Carotenoids. *Journal of Pharmacognosy and Phytochemistry, 2*, 225-234.

Elliott, R. (2005). Mechanisms of genomic and non-genomic actions of carotenoids. *Biochimica et Biophysica Acta, 1740,* 147-154.

El-Qudah, J. M. (2008). Dietary intake of selected common vegetable foods and their total carotenoids determination. *American Journal of Agricultural and Biological Sciences*, *3*, 729-733.

Fiedor, J. and Burda, K. (2014). Potential role of carotenoids as antioxidants in human health and disease. *Nutrients, 6*, 466-488.

Finkel, T. and Holbrook, N. J. (2000). Oxidants, oxidative stress and the biology of aging. *Nature, 408*, 239-247.

Fraser, P. D. and Bramley, P. M. (2004). The biosynthesis and nutritional uses of carotenoids. *Progress in Lipid Research*, *43*, 228-265.

Gärtner, C., Stahl, W., Sies, H. (1997). Lycopene is more biovailable from tomato paste than from fresh tomatoes. *American Journal of Clinical Nutrition, 66,* 116-122.

Giovannucci, E. (2005). Tomato products, lycopene, and prostate cancer: a review of the epidemiological literature. *Journal of Nutrition, 135*, 2030-2031S.

Giovannucci, E. (1999). Tomatoes, tomato-based products, lycopene, and cancer: review of the epidemiologic literature. *Journal of the National Cancer Institute, 91*, 317-333.

Gul, K., Tak, A., Singh, A. K., Singh, P., Yousuf, B., Wani, A. A. (2015). Chemistry, encapsulation, and health benefits of β-carotene- A review. *Cogent Food and Agriculture, 1*, 1-12.

Hadley, C. W., Clinton, S. K., Schwartz, S. J. (2003). The consumption of processed tomato products enhances plasma lycopene concentrations in association with a reduced lipoprotein sensitivity to oxidative damage. *Journal of Nutrition, 133,* 727-732.

Halliwell, B. and Gutteridge, J. M. C. (1999). *Free radicals in biology and medicine* (3rd ed.). Oxford, UK: Oxford University Press.

Hänsch, R. and Mendel, R. R. (2009). Physiological functions of mineral micronutrients (Cu, Zn, Mn, Fe, Ni, Mo, B, Cl). *Current Opinion in Plant Biology*, *12*, 259-266.

Haskell, M. J. (2012). The challengue to reach nutritional adequacy for vitamin A: β-carotene bioavailability and conversion-evidence in humans. *American Journal of Clinical Nutrition, 96*, 1193S-1203S.

Hennekens, C. H., Buring, J. E., Manson, J. E., Stampfer, M., Rosner, B., Cook, N. R., Belanger, C., LaMotte, F., Gaziano, J. M., Ridker, P. M., Willet, W., Peto, R. (1996). Lack of effect of long-term supplementation with beta carotene on the incidence of malignant neoplasms and cardiovascular disease. *New England Journal Medicine, 334*, 1145-1149.

Het-Hof, K. H., West, C. E., Wetstrate, J. A., Hautvast, J. G. (2005). Dietary factors that affect the bioavailability of carotenoids. *Journal of Nutrition, 130*, 503-506.

Jain, C. K., Agarwal, S., Rao, A. V. (1999). The effect of dietary lycopene on bioavailability, tissue distribution, in-vivo antioxidant properties and colonic preneoplasia in rats. *Nutrition Research, 19*, 1383-1391.

Jaswir, I., Noviendri, D., Hasrini, R. F., Octavianti, F. (2011). Carotenoids: Sources, medicinal properties and their application in food and nutraceutical industry. *Journal of Medicinal Plants Research, 5*, 7119-7131.

Kalt, W. (2005). Effects of production and processing factor on major fruit and vegetable antioxidants. *Journal of Food Science, 70*, R11-R19.

Khachik, F. (2006). Distribution and metabolism of dietary carotenoids in humans as a criterion for developments of nutritional supplements. *Pure and Applied Chemistry, 78*, 1551-1557.

Krinsky, N. I. (1998). Overview of lycopene, carotenoids, and disease prevention. *Proceeding of the Society for Experimental Biology and Medicine, 218*, 95-97.

Le-Marchand, L., Hankin, J. H., Kolonel, L. N., Beecher, C. R., Wilkens, L. R., Zhao, L. P. (1993). Intake of specific carotenoids and lung cancer risk. *Cancer Epidemiology Biomarkers and Prevention, 2*, 182-187.

Liu, R. H. (2007). Whole grain phytochemicals and health. *Journal of Cereal Science, 46*, 207-219.

Margalith, P. Z. (1999). Production of ketocarotenoids by microalgae. *Applied Microbiology and Biotechnology, 51,* 431-438.

Martin, K. R., Failla, M. L., Smith, J. C. (1996). Beta-carotene and lutein protect HepG2 human liver cells against oxidant-induced damage. *Journal of Nutrition, 126*, 2098-2106.

Maughan, R. (2005). Basic metabolism II: Carbohydrate. *Surgery (Oxford), 23*, 154-158.

Mayne, S. T. (1996). Beta-carotene, carotenoids, and disease preventions in humans. *FASEB Journal, 10*, 690-701.

Melendez-Martinez, A. J., Vicario, I. M., Heredia, J. (2004). Stability of carotenoid pigments in foods. *Archivos Latinoamericanos de nutrición, 54,* 2009-2015.

Mohanty, I., Joshi, S., Trivedi, D., Srivastava, S., Gupta, S. K. (2002). Lycopene prevents sugar-induced morphological changes and modulates antioxidant status of human lens epithelial cells. *British Journal of Nutrition, 88*, 347-354.

Nahum, A., Hirsch, K., Danilenko, M., Watts, C. K. W., Prall, O. W. J., Levy, J., Sharoni, Y. (2001). Lycopene inhibition of cell cycle progression in breast and endometrial cancer cells associated with reduction in cyclin D levels en retention of p^{27KipI} in the cyclin E-cdk2 complexes. *Oncogene, 20,* 3428-3436.

Ndolo, V. U. and Beta, T. (2013). Distribution of carotenoids in endosperm, germ, and aleurone fractions of cereal grain kernesl. *Food Chemistry, 139*, 663-671.

Olson, J. A. (1994). Absorption, transport, and metabolism of carotenoids in humans. *Pure and Applied Chemistry, 66*, 1011-1016.

Parker, R. S. (1988). Carotenoid and tocopherol composition in human adipose tissue. *American Journal of Clinical Nutrition, 47,* 33-36.

Prabhashankar-Arathi, B., Raghavendra-Rao, P., Sowmya, Vijay, K., Baskaran, V., Lakshminarayana, R. (2015). Metabolomics of carotenoids:

The challenges and prospect. *Treds in Food Science and Technology*, *45,* 105-117.

Qian, C., Decker, E. A., Xiao, H., McClements, D. J. (2012). Physical and chemical stability of β-carotene-enriched nanoemulsions: Influence of pH, ionic strength, temperature, and emulsifier type. *Food Chemistry*, *132*, 1221-1229.

Rao, A. V. and Rao, L. G. (2007). Carotenoids and human health. *Pharmacological Research*, *55*, 207-216.

Rodriguez-Amaya, D. and Kimura, M. (2004). *HarvestPlus Handbook of Carotenoid Analysis* (1rs ed.). Washington, DC: HarvestPlus.

Sindhu, E. R., Preethi, K. C., Kuttan, R. (2010). Antioxidant activity of carotenoid lutein *in vitro* and *in vivo*. *Indian Journal of Experimental Biology*, *48*, 843-848.

Singh, P. and Goyal, G. K. (2008). Dietary lycopene: Its properties and anticarcinogenic effects. *Comprehensive Reviews in Food Science and Food Safety*, *7*, 255-270.

Smigel, K. (1990). Beta-carotene didn´t prevent cancer: what´s up, doc? *Journal of the National Cancer Institute, 82*, 899-900.

Stadtman, E. R. (2004). Role of oxidant species in aging. *Current Medical Chemistry, 11,* 1105-1112.

Stahl, W. and Sies, H. (1992). Uptake of lycopene and its geometrical isomers is greater from heat-processed than from unprocessed tomato juice in humans. *Journal of Nutrition*, *122,* 2161-2166.

Stahl, W. and Sies, H. (2005). Bioactivity and protective effects of natural carotenoids. *Biochimica et Biophysica Acta*, *1740,* 101-107.

Summerburg, O., Keunen, J. E. E., Bird, A. C., van Kuijk, F. J. G. M. (1998). Fruits and vegetables that are sources for lutein and zeaxanthin: the macular pigment in human eyes. *British Journal of Ophthalmology, 82*, 907-910.

Tanaka, T., Shnimizu, M., Moriwaki, H. (2012). Cancer chemoprevention by carotenoids. *Molecules*, *17,* 3202-3242.

Truscott, T. G. (1990). The photophysics and photochemistry of the carotenoids. *Journal of Photochemistry and Photobiology B: Biology, 6,* 359-371.

Valko, M., Leibfritz, D., Moncol, J., Cronin, M. T. D., Mazur, M., Telser, J. (2007). Free radicals and antioxidants in normal physiological functions and human disease. *The International Journal of Biochemistry and Cell Biology, 39*, 44-84.

Valko, M., Rhodes, C. J., Moncol, J., Izakovic, M., Mazur, M. (2006). Free radicals, metals and antioxidants in oxidative stress-induced cancer. *Chemico-Biological Interactions, 160*, 1-40.

van Breeman, R. B., Xu, X., Viana, M. A., Chen, L., Stacewicz-Sapuntzakis, M., Duncan, C., Bowen, P. E., Sharifi, R. (2002). Liquid chromatography-mass spectrometry of cis-and all-trans-lycopene in human serum and prostate tissue after dietary supplementation with tomato sauce. *Journal of Agricultural and Food Chemistry, 50*, 2214-2219.

van Poppel, G. (1993). Carotenoids and cancer: and update with emphasis on human intervention studies. *European Journal of Cancer, 29*, 1335-1344.

van Poppel, G. and Goldbohom, R. A. (1995). Epidemiologic evidence for beta-carotene and cancer prevention. *American Journal of Clinical Research, 62,* 1393S-1402S.

Vogiatzi, G., Tousoulis, D., Stefanadis, C. (2009). The role of oxidative stress in aterosclerosis. *Hellenic Journal of Cardiology, 50,* 402-409.

Voutilainen, S., Nurmi, T., Mursu, J., Rissanen, T. H. (2006). Carotenoids and cardiovascular health. *American Journal Clinical Nutrition, 83*, 1265-1271.

Williams, A. W., Boileau, T. W., Erdman, J. W. (1998). Factors influencing the uptake and absorption of carotenoids. *Experimental Biology and Medicine, 218*, 106-108.

Wurtzel, E., Cuttriss, A. J., Vallabhaneni, R. (2012). Maize provitamin A carotenoids current resources and future metabolic engineering challenges. *Frontiers in Plant Science, 3*, 1-12.

Yahia, E. M. and Ornelas-Paz, J. J. (2010). Chemistry, stability, and biological actions of carotenoids. In: de la Rosa, L. A., Alvarez-Padilla, E., Gonzalez-Aguilar, G. A., editors. *Fruit and Vegetable Phytochemicals*: *Chemistry, Nutritional value, and Stability* (1rs ed., pp. 177-222). Ames, Iowa: Wiley-Blackwell.

Young, A. J. and Lowe, G. M. (2001). Antioxidant and prooxidant properties of carotenoids. *Archives of Biochemistry and Biophysics, 385*, 20-27.

In: Carotenoids
Editors: Hanne Leif and Felix Ulrik
ISBN: 978-1-53612-685-3

Chapter 2

Carotenoids in Microalgae

Andrêssa S. Fernandes, Pricila N. Pinheiro, Mariany C. Deprá, Eduardo Jacob-Lopes and Leila Q. Zepka

Department of Food Science and Technology,
Federal University of Santa Maria (UFSM), Santa Maria, RS, Brazil

Abstract

The carotenoids are isoprenoids, highly unsatured, lipophilic, featuring a variety cores from yellow to red. Appoximately 750 naturally occurring, and many of this tetraterpenes are produced from microalgae. The composition of carotenoids from microalgae can still be complex, with structural characteristics very different from those commonly found in foods, such as a greater number of carbon atoms, of c.d.b., and of hydroxyl groups, which all contribute to their great antioxidant capacity. These compounds have properties that result in biological functions beneficial to human health, such as cellular protection against free radicals, it is know that the antioxidant properties of the carotenoids are are closely related to their chemical structure. Carotenoids are a source of several bioactive compounds with great otential for applications in food, cosmect, and pharmaceutical industries. Thus, the chapter is organized in three major topics. (1) fundamental aspects of structure and biosynthesis of carotenoids from microalgae, (2) bioactive carotenoids from microalgae, (3) examples of novelty to industrial applications.

Keywords: microalgae, biosynthesis, pigments, biotechnology.

INTRODUCTION

Microalgae are fast growing organisms which produce a variety of compounds which have various commercial uses them to the synthesis of bioactive compounds like pigments, and vitamins [1].

In addition, microalgae have always Been Considered the typical of photosynthetic microorganisms in the CO_2 fixing dependent light is the dominant mode of nutrition [2]. Also can be grown heterotrophically, without light and with addition of an exogenous carbon source using the pentose phosphate pathway. Such metabolic route serves as a source for obtaining the carotenoid biosynthetic precursors which can be divided into five main steps. The initial stages consist of formation of isopentenyl diphosphate (IPP) and the chain elongation to geranygeranyl diphosphate (GGPP) and formation of phytoene [3].

Consuming carotenoid has been widely associated with beneficial health effects, is mainly attributed to its antioxidant properties. The imbalance between the generation of reactive oxygen species (ROS) and antioxidant status can lead to oxidative stress, which is implicated in the pathology of chronic degenerative diseases and aging processes [4].

In view of the commercial importance of these pigments the objective of the chapter this was to elucidate the fundamental aspects of structure, biosynthesis and bioactive of carotenoids from microalgae and industrial applications.

BIOSYNTHESIS OF CAROTENOIDS IN MICROALGAE

Most microalgae groups possess two cellular isoprenoid biosynthesis pathways as higher plants: the mevalonic acid (MVA) pathway for biosynthesis of the cytosolic sterols and the methylerythritol phosphate (MEP) pathway [5, 6, 7, 8, 9] present in the plastids of plants occurring in all studied microalgae species from all classes [8, 9, 10, 11].

In general, microalgae are commonly grown by fixing dissolved, inorganic carbon (CO2) and absorbing solar energy. Therefore, like most land-based plants, they perform photosynthesis and are photo-autotrophs. At the same time, some species of microalgae are also heterotrophic, using organic compounds in the growth medium as carbon and energy sources therefore, they do not need light as an energy source [12, 13].

The Figure 1 demonstrate the scheme the biosynthesis direct precursors methylerythritol phosphatethe (MEP) pathway, the glyceraldehyde 3-phosphate (GAP) and pyruvate, cultivation photoautotrophic in which CO2 and light energy are used as the carbon and energy sources, respectively [14], form Calvin cycle CO2 is rapidly transformed to 3-phosphoglyceric acid (3-PGA) and reduced to glyceraldehyde-3-phosphate (GAP) [5, 15]. Pyruvate directly from photosynthetically fixed carbon via 3-phosphoglyceric acid (3-PGA) and phosphoenol pyruvate (PEP) [5, 16, 17].

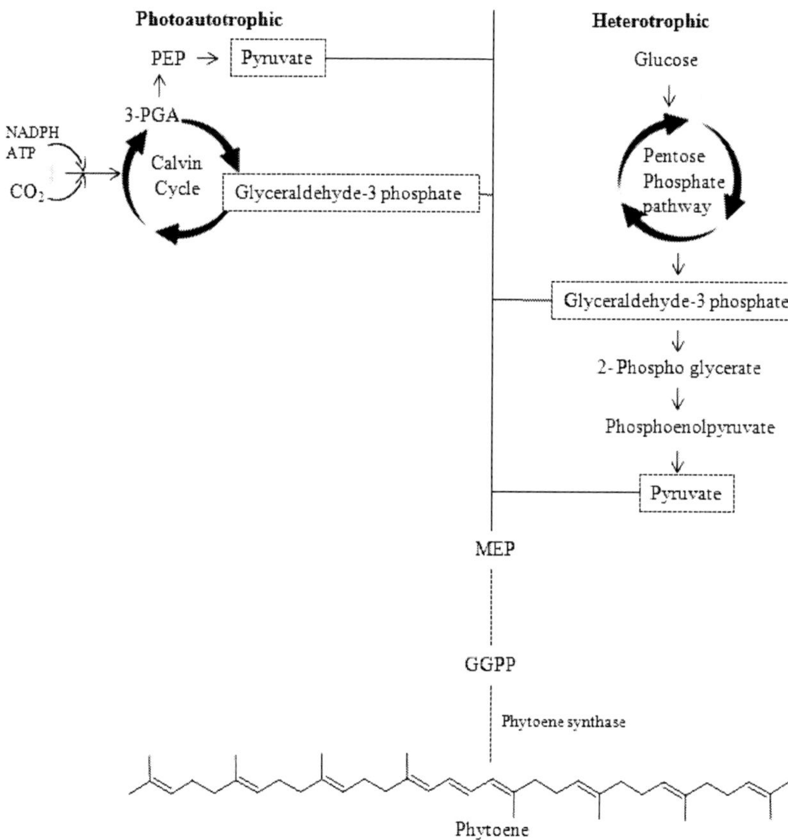

Figure 1. The biosynthesis direct precursors methylerythritol phosphate (MEP) pathway, the glyceraldehyde 3-phosphate (GAP) and pyruvate, in cultivation photoautotrophic the heterotrophic. 3-PGA= 3-phosphoglyceric acid; respectively; PEP= phosphoenolpyruvate; GGPP= geranygeranyl diphosphate.

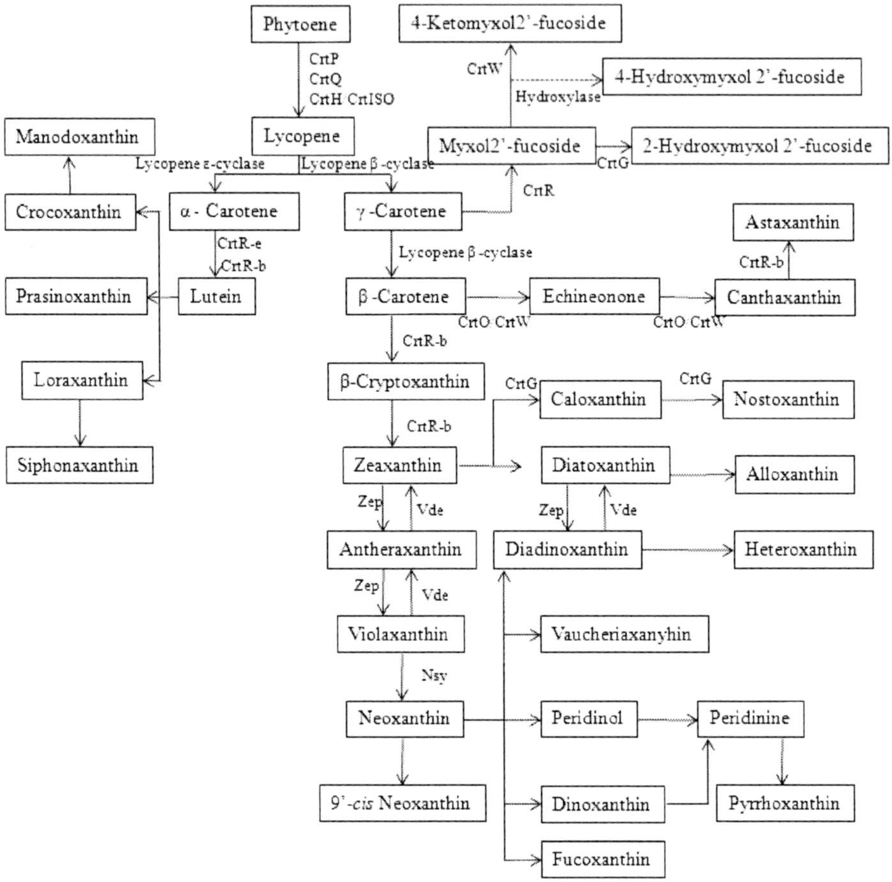

Figure 2. Diagram of pathway of carotenoids biosynthesis.

Although pigments are traditionally thought to be the outcome of metabolisms associated with exposure to light, the capacity of some microalgae to produce some of them in the dark under specific growth conditions opens a line of research that is barely explored [18]. In cultivation heterotrophic the assimilation of one or more organic substrates as the carbon is through the Pentose Phosphate pathway has been found in microalgae [12, 19]. The glucose preferred substrate because it is utilized by a broader range of organisms as a sole carbon source and easily gives rise to the precursors for both isoprenoid biosynthetic routes [7, 20]. These glucose catabolic routes yield glyceraldehyde 3-phosphate (GAP) and pyruvate; which are the two precursors in the MEP pathway.

Synthesized by either the two pathways the geranylgeranyl diphosphate (GGPP), the isopentenyl diphosphate (IPP) is isomerized to its allylic isomer, dimethylallyl diphosphate (DMAPP). Geranyl pyrophosphate (GPP) is then produced by the condensation reaction of IPP and DMAPP elongation of GPP by the addition of IPP results in the formation of farnesyl pyrophosphate (FPP) to which is further added another IPP to produce GGPP [14, 21]. In a head-to-head condensation of the two GGPP C20 compounds, the first carotene phytoene (C40).

Microalgae require three enzymes in the conversion from phytoene to lycopene: phytoene desaturase (CrtP), δ-carotene desaturase (CrtQ) and cis-carotene isomerase (CrtH), all carotenoids microalgae are derived from lycopene: β-carotene, α-carotene and their derivatives [22]. Exceptionally in cyanobacteria can synthesize some unique types of carotenoids, myxol glycosides and oscillol diglycosides are monocyclic and acyclic carotenoids respectively (Figure 2) [22, 23].

Bioactive Carotenoids and Their Properties Physiological

Among the bioproducts of microalgae with possible bioactive properties, there is great interest in naturally occurring pigments, which is highlighted carotenoids due to its unique properties and its potential beneficial effects on human health, such as provitamin A, antioxidants, anti-inflammatory, anti-tumor and anti-cancer, thus showing potential exploitation as bioactive compounds [23, 24, 25, 26, 27], these classified as phytochemicals capable of modulating metabolic processes essential to the health of the cells, due to their protective action on the cellular components against oxidative damage [28, 29].

The carotenoids consist of a symmetrical structure with a set of conjugated double bonds (c.d.b), called the chromophore absorbing light, this part of the structure responsible for the color and the properties and special features [3], such as a high antioxidant capacity [30]. Therefore, most bioactive capacity carotenoid microalgae is directly related bathochromic effect that occurs in these structures. In order that the antioxidant activity of the compounds increases directly with the increase of chromophore. However, the chain elongation also renders the molecule susceptible to geometric isomerization and oxidative degradation [3, 31].

Consequently, microalgae are able to synthesize a wide range of structural variety, where some of these compounds have diverse structures of other carotenoids found in nature. Among the carotenoids from the microalgae important role in the bioactivity level is the β-carotene, a predominant carotenoid in the group of carotenes to be composed only of carbon and hydrogen atoms. In parallel, microalgae are also able to synthesize xanthophylls, carotenoids consist of at least one oxygen atom. The major carotenoids in microalgae have reported are β-carotene, their hydroxy derivatives, zeaxanthin, its keto derivative, echinenone, lutein, canthaxanthin, antheraxanthin, violaxanthin, astaxanthin and mixo xantophil [23, 32, 33, 34, 35]. Carotenoids these, which stands out in terms of power of synthesis and have a higher bioactive capacity.

Numerous algae have shown the ability to synthesis of carotenoids, some are listed in Table 1. In recent work described by Rodrigues [23], was possible to identify the microalgae extract Phormidium showed the presence of characteristic ketocarotenoids and glycosylated carotenoids in cyanobacteria such as all-trans canthaxanthin (0.93 ug.g-1), all-trans-myxoxanthophyll (3.15 ug.g-1), all-trans-echinenone (19.87 ug.g-1) and cis-echinenone (15.70 ug.g-1) and due to their singular antioxidant properties and their potential beneficial effects on human health these carotenoids show potential of exploration like bioactive compounds. In work described by Goiris [36], emphasized that the carotenoid content from microalgae is that the upper end is obtained by conventional sources, while xanthophylls are found in higher proportion. Among these carotenoids from microalgae are the main β-carotene, lutein, violaxanthin, zeaxanthin, astaxanthin, and neoxantina to be carotenoid that stand out in terms of power of synthesizing these microorganisms and present a greater bioactive capacity [22, 23, 36, 37, 38, 39, 40]. All of these compounds in fact, fall into the class of xanthophylls by having oxygen in its structure, except the β-carotene which is absent in this compound.

It is suggested a higher antioxidant activity for microalgal carotenoids when compared to conventional sources because of the presence of unique carotenoids, which exhibit bathochromic effect, as is the case with the equinenona and cataxantina chromophore of 12 and 13 respectively (c.d.b) [41, 42], it is known that the extension of the chromophore is closely linked to increased antioxidant activity.

In addition to being potent antioxidants some carotenoids activity pro vitamin A [43]. In all existing carotenoids, only 10% exhibit provitamin A activity. Among the most important, both for its high level of activity than their availability, are α- and β-carotene, and xanthophylls including some β-cryptoxanthin and some apocarotenoids [44].

However, only those with at least one ring of the β type without oxygenated functional groups with a chain polyene having at least 11 carbon atoms are potential precursors of vitamin A. Of these, β-carotene has the highest provitamin A activity since each retinal pigment molecule produces two, which is then reduced to vitamin a (retinol) [45].

In man, the conversion of beta-carotene to vitamin A is catalysed by the cleavage of the carotenoids (mainly at the intestine) by the enzymeβ-carotene 15,15′-dioxygenase.

Antioxidant Activities

Various reactive species oxygens are generated continuously by our metabolism ($1O_2$, OH•, O_2 •- ROO•, e H_2O_2), addition also takes place exogenous sources of free radicals (for example radiation, tobacco smoke and pesticides) which human beings are exposed [46]. They are damaging biologically important molecules like lipids, DNA or proteins and are involved in the pathobiochemistry of degenerative diseases [47].

Among the various defense strategies, carotenoids are most likely involved in the scavenging of two of the reactive oxygen species, singlet molecular oxygen ($1O_2$), and peroxyl radicals [47].

Carotenoids have bioactive properties primarily due to the excellent physical Quenching singlet oxygen ($1O_2$), where the energy absorbed paragraph produce triplet oxygen ($3O_2$) is converted to rotary and vibratory energy by the chromophore system carotenoid, as well as potent scavengers of other reactive oxygen species (ROS) [46, 48, 49, 50]. The quenching rate of carotenoids increases with increasing numbers of double bounds and varies with functional groups and chain structure [3].

Several studies have reviewed antioxidant actions of carotenoids, but the role of antioxidant for carotenoid is still complex, because these compounds show a pro-oxidant effect which occurs in a high concentration of oxygen in the medium or carotenoids, although this information is still controversial and you cannot distract from their health benefits [46, 51].

Table 1. Carotenoids in Microalgae

Compounds	Microalgae	Reference
β-caroteno; echinenone; cantaxanthin	*Phormidium sp.*	Rodrigues et al, 2015 [23]
β-caroteno	*Dunaliella salina*	El-Baz et al., 2002 [67]
β-caroteno, lutein	*Dunaliella salina*	García-González et al., 2005 [44]
Astaxanthin	*Chlorella zofingiensis*	Ip & Chen, 2005 [38]
Astaxanthin	*Chlorella zofingiensis* *Haematococcus pluvialis*	Han & Hu, 2013 [39]
Astaxanthin	*Chlorella; Haematococcus*	Kim, et al., 2016 [40]
Lutein	*Chlorella sorokiniana*	Chen, et al., 2016 [37]
Zeaxanthin; neoxanthin, violaxanthin; lutein; β-caroteno; antheraxanthin	*Chlorella protothecoides; Chlorella vulgaris*	Grudzinski et al., 2016 [68]
Astaxanthin	*Haematococcus pluvialis*	Panis & Carreon, 2016 [69]
Lutein	*Coelastrella sp.; Desmodesmus sp*	Chiu, Soong & Chen, 2016 [70]
Canthaxanthin; echinenone;	*Scenedesmus sp.*	Abrahamsson, Rodriguez-Meizoso & Turner, 2012 [71]
β-caroteno; lutein	*Chlorella salina*	Gayathri et al., 2016 [72]
Neoxanthin; lutein; β-caroteno; astaxanthin,	*Haematococcus pluvialis*	Jaime et al., 2010 [73]

Cantaxanthin; astaxanthin; lutein	*Chlamydocapsa spp*	Leya et al., 2009 [74]

The antioxidant properties of carotenoids are associated with their radical scavenging properties and their exceptional ability of singlet oxygen ($1O_2$) quenching [51]. These compounds are very potent natural antioxidants because of their energy levels and their $1O_2$ quenching process, which proves to be very effective, especially for carotenoid containing 11 or more conjugated double bonds [48].

In general, the overall process oxygen deactivating singlet $1O_2$ for carotenoid is based on converting excess energy to heat through lower carotenoid [CAR] for triplet excited state [3CAR] [48, 51, 49]. This process is represented in the equation below.

$$1O2 + [CAR] \rightarrow 3O2 + [3CAR]$$
$$[3CAR] \rightarrow [CAR] + heat$$

According El-Agamey [51] and Rodrigues-Amaya [3], carotenoids [CAR] may scavenge radicals in an initial step that involves one or more of the following three possibilities (namely, electron transfer, allylic hydrogen abstraction) represented in the following equation:

$$[CAR] + ROO\bullet \rightarrow [CAR]\bullet+ + ROO- \text{ (Electron transfer)}$$
$$[CAR] + ROO\bullet \rightarrow [CAR]\bullet + ROOH \text{ (Hydrogen abstraction)}$$
$$[CAR] + ROO\bullet \rightarrow [ROOCAR]\bullet \text{ (Addition)}$$

The factors that may influence the antioxidant activity of carotenoids in biological systems are (I) the structure and physical form of the carotenoid molecule, (II) the location or site of action of the carotenoid molecule within the cell, (III) the potential for interaction with other carotenoids or antioxidants (especially vitamins C and E), (IV) the concentration of the carotenoid, and (V) the partial pressure of oxygen [3].

Rodrigues [23], identified in the study with the microalgae Phormidium sp. 20 different carotenoids, and all-trans-β-carotene, 13-cis-zeaxanthin, all-trans-lutein, all-trans-canthaxanthin and all-trans-echinenone represent the carotenoids class (xanthophylls) having a greater number conjugated double bonds at its structure, thus causing, expansion of the chromophore which provides higher carotenoid antioxidant power.

Research is being conducted with astaxanthin from microalgae as a potent antioxidant to human health [39]. In particular, studies have reported that the antioxidant properties of astaxanthin are about 10 times higher than those of β-carotene, lutein, zeaxanthin, canthaxanthin and more than 500 times greater than α-tocopherol [52, 53]. In studies conducted by Yamashita [54], it was possible to identify this pigment in the species of microalgae and you realize that is about 40 times more potent than that of β-carotene in singlet oxygen quenching. Other works also demonstrate the presence of astaxanthin, lutein in canthaxanthin in microalgae [55].

Several studies have shown that carotenoids interact synergistically with several other antioxidants. The best known example is probably between beta-carotene and alpha-tocopherol (vitamin E) in the protection of in vivo lipid peroxidation. Another example, however, is zeaxanthin in combination with ascorbic acid (vitamin C) and vitamin E, which, together protecting human retinal pigment cells against oxidation reactions induced photoreactions [46].

BIOAVAILABILITY AND BIOACCESSIBILITY OF CAROTENOIDS

Before carotenoids can perform their health-promoting functions, they have to reach their sites of action. They must be absorbed from the intestine, transported in the circulation, and delivered to target tissues. These complicated processes are subject to many influencing factors [3].

Bioavailability refers to the portion of the carotenoid which is absorbed in the body, enters in systemic circulation and becomes available for utilization in normal physiological functions or for storage in the human body [3]. May be affected by a number of factors such as: the complexity of the matrix; chemical structure of the substance of interest; structure and amount of other compounds in the diet as well as the mass of the mucosa and intestinal transit time; the rate of gastric emptying; metabolism and the degree of conjugation and bond with carrier proteins in blood and tissues [56].

Therefore, it is known bioactive compounds that only become bioavailable in the body after being released from the food matrix and modified in the gastrointestinal tract [29]. Consequently, the bioavailable amount, which is responsible for the beneficial effects on health, antioxidant and anti-inflammatory for example, always differ from the original contents of the array, since the bioactive compounds undergo changes during the digestion process. However, it has been shown that the bioavailability of carotenoids in fruits and vegetables is significantly lower than that of algae-derived supplements [57].

According Carbonnel Capella [29], different approaches to study the bioaccessibility and bioavailability of bioactive compounds include in vitro methods (simulating gastrointestinal digestion, artificial membranes, Caco-2 cell cultures, isolation/reconstitution membranes, Ussing chambers), ex vivo techniques (gastrointestinal organs in laboratory conditions), in situ tests (intestinal perforation in animals) and in vivo models (in human and animal studies).

Bioavailability is best determined through human studies; bioaccessibility has been widely evaluated in vitro [3]. Bohn [58], describes various techniques to check the bioavailability of carotenoids.

Both in vitro tests and in vivo have advantages and disadvantages. In in vitro tests the main advantages relate to relatively inexpensive and simple techniques and uptake when followed by Caco-2 epithelial cell absorption is similar to standard conditions [59]. The main disadvantage is the extrapolation stop living in, because the conditions of the gastrointestinal tract are not fully reproduced. In in vivo tests the actual condition of digestion is the main advantage, the major challenge is the ethical constraint and lack of certificates procedure, moreover, is the extrapolation from animal studies to humans.

With reference to bioavailability studies microalgal of carotenoids, these are limited because pretreatment extract purification before the intake of these compounds is necessary in order compounds which may have toxic to human health.

INDUSTRIAL APPLICATIONS

The great interest in microalgae cultivation is the metabolite production capacity with high industrial value extracted from the biomass [1, 60]. Among these compounds includes the pigments, once which microalgae are recognized as an excellent source of carotenoids [25].

Bioactive pigments, such as extract carotenoids can be obtained by different extraction techniques. However, studies have been elucidated in order to develop methodologies involving non-toxic extraction methods related to green chemistry and renewable biological resources that are economically viable for production on an industrial scale.

In a process of extraction, the toxicity of the solvents used, the degradation of the compounds and the selectivity of the method are major points must be considered. When produced biologically, the pigments promote an exponential demand in the industrial market, the extent to which the availability for biotech companies provide benefits such as cost and ease of production will become an important source the competition of bioproduction with chemical synthesis. In addition, the parameters that should be considered include (1) the source of these bioactive compounds, in this case, microalgae; (2) yield obtained in a given process of extraction; (3) productivity; and (4) the selectivity [61].

There are plenty of methods to obtain carotenoid extracts. Among the most used are solvents, acids, edible oils, supercritical fluids, assisted by microwave assisted enzyme and approaches. However, when considered more efficient and compatible methods include the solvents but supercritical fluids such as carbon dioxide (SC-CO_2) are the most used by industries in the economic viability regard [62].

The production of carotenoids using microalgae as feedstock has become one of the most successful activities in the biotechnology industry [63]. When industrially applied the carotenoids are widely used as color enhancers in natural foods including egg yolk, chicken meat or fish. On the face of it, the use of natural colorants has been steadily increasing primarily because of changes in consumer preference toward more natural products known to exhibit specific functional properties [64].

Currently, German chemical company - BASF is the undisputed world leader in beta-carotene production from Dunaliella salina, with over a thousand hectares of production ponds in two plants in Australia [24]. Consequently, due to this increased demand for pigments the β-carotene, the global market of carotenoids, is estimated to 2016 the value at USD 1.24 Billion. Furthermore, the prospects indicate in 2021 the value projected for USD $ 1.53 billion [65].

Additionally, the major market for astaxanthin is the production of Haematococcus spp, known by the great accumulation of astaxanthin, the pigment responsible for the pinkish-red applied to the flesh of salmonids and other sources obtained by aquaculture. Other commercial ways of these pigments are in the form of the capsule, soft gel, tablet, powder, biomass, cream, energy drink, oil and extract. According to Cysewski [66], It is estimated that the value of astaxanthin in the world market can reach US $ 200 million, making the astaxanthin carotenoid another of the high value produced from microalgae commercial.

Some carotenoids derived specifically from microalgae as echinenone have a promising economic appeal, once 1 mg echinenone is currently sold on the market per RS 3,345.00 [42]. In addition, one of the advantages of industrial application of microalgae is that many other antioxidant compounds present in biomass are transported along with these pigments providing a synergistic effect and consequently the positive impact on human health.

Finally, the bioactive compounds synthesized by microalgae are of major importance to the industrial market. However, the use of microalgae as a source of carotenoids bioactives compounds to promote antioxidant activity, remains questionable due to many factors has not been completely clarified, and the instability of these compounds and the study of their bioavailability. In this regard, the extent to which the biosynthesis of these structures from microalgae are elucidated application will be useful in industries. In business view, efforts should be made to consolidate the technological process of producing the same.

REFERENCES

[1] Dufossé, L. (2016). *Current and Potential Natural Pigments From Microorganisms (Bacteria, Yeasts, Fungi, Microalgae).*

[2] Fay, P. (1983). *The blue-greens (Cyanophyta – Cyanobacteria)* (5th Ed.), Great Britain.

[3] Rodriguez-Amaya, D.B. (2016). Food Carotenoids: Chemistry, Biology and Technology, Pondichery.

[4] Del Campo, J.A.; García-Gonzáles, M.; Guerrero, M.G. (2007). Outdoor cultivation of microalgae for carotenoid production: current state and perspectives. *Applied microbiology biotechnology*, 74, 1163-1174.

[5] Lichtenthaler, H.K. (2010). *The Chloroplast: Basics and Applications.* (8th Ed.), Dordrecht.

[6] Lichtenthaler, H.K. (1999). The 1-deoxy- D -xylulose-5-phosphate pathway of isoprenoid biosynthesis in plants. *Annual Review of Plant Physiology and Plant Molecular Biology*; 50: 47–65.

[7] Disch, A.; Schwender, J.; Müller, C.; Lichtenthaler, H.K.; Rohmer, M. (1998). Distribution of the mevalonate and glyceraldehyde phosphate/pyruvate pathways for isoprenoid biosynthesis in unicellular algae and the cyanobacterium Synechocystis PCC 6714. *Biochemical Journal*; 333:381–388.

[8] Lichtenthaler, H.K.; Schwender, J.; Disch, A.; Rohmer, M. (1997). Biosynthesis of isoprenoids in higher plant chloroplasts proceeds via a mevalonate independent pathway. *FEBS Letters*; 400: 271–274.

[9] Schwender, J.; Zeidler, J.; Gröner, R.; Müller, C.; Focke, M.; Braun, S.; Lichtenthaler; F.W.; Lichtenthaler, H.K. (1997). Incorporation of 1-

deoxy-d-xylulose into isoprene and phytol by higher plants and algae. *FEBS Letters*; 414: 129–134.

[10] Egeland, E.S. (2016). *The Physiology of Microalgae*. (3th Ed.), Switzerland.

[11] Lohr, M.; Schwender, J.; Polle, J.E.W. (2012). Isoprenoid biosynthesis in eukaryotic phototrophs: a spotlight on algae. *Plant Science*; 186: 9–22.

[12] Perez-Garcia, O.; Bashan, Y. (2015). *Algal biorefineries II: products and biorefinery design*. (3th Ed.), Switzerland.

[13] Chen, G.Q.; Chen, F. (2006). Growing phototrophic cells without light. *Biotechnology Letters*; 28: 607–616.

[14] Sun, Z.; Li, T.; Zhou, Z.; Jiang, Y. (2015). *Microalgae Biotechnology*. (2th Ed.), Switzerland.

[15] Calvin, M.; Bassham, J.A. (1962). *The Photosynthesis of Carbon Compounds*, New York.

[16] Schulze-Siebert, D.; Schulze, G. (1987). ß-carotene synthesis in isolated chloroplasts. *Plant Physiology*; 84: 1233–1237.

[17] Schulze-Siebert, D.; Heinecke, D.; Scharf, H.; Schulze, G. (1984). Pyruvate-derived amino acids in spinach chloroplasts. *Plant Physiology*; 76: 465–471.

[18] Perez-Garcia, O.; Escalante, F.M.E.; de-Bashan, L.E.; Bashan, Y. (2011). Heterotrophic cultures of microalgae: metabolism and potential products. *Water Research*; 45: 11–36.

[19] Neilson, A.H.; Lewin, R.A. (1974). The uptake and utilization of organic carbon by algae: an essay in comparative biochemistry. *Phycologia*; 13: 227–264.

[20] Eisenreich, W.; Bacher, A.; Arigoni, D.; Rohdich, F. (2004). Biosynthesis of isoprenoids via the non-mevalonate pathway. *Cellular and Molecular Life Sciences*; 61: 1401–1426.

[21] Fraser, P.D.; Schuch, W.; Bramley, P.M. (2000). Phytoene synthase from tomato (Lycopersicon esculentum) chloroplasts-partial purification and biochemical properties. *Planta* 211, 361–369.

[22] Takaichi, S. (2011) Carotenoids in algae: distributions, biosyntheses and functions. *Marine Drugs*, 9, 1101-1118.

[23] Rodrigues, D.R.; Flores, E.M.M.; Barin, J.S.; Mercadante, A.Z.; Jacob-Lopes, E.; Zepka, L.Q. (2014). Production of carotenoids from microalgae cultivated using agroindustrial wastes. *Food Research International*, 65, 144-148.

[24] Borowitzka, M. A. (2013). High-value products from microalgae-their development and commercialization. *Journal of Applied Phycology*, 25, 743-756.

[25] Maadane, A.; Merghouba N.; Hicham, A.; Arroussi, E.; Benhimaa, R.; Amzazib, S.; Bakrib, Y.; Wahbya, I. (2015). Antioxidant activity of some Moroccan marine microalgae: Pufa profiles, carotenoids and phenolic content. *Journal of Biotechnology*, 215, 13-19.

[26] Guedes, A.C.; Amaro, H.M.; Malcata, F.X. (2011). Microalgae as sources of carotenoids. *Marine Drugs*, 9, 625–644.

[27] Ho, N. H.; Inbaraj, B. S.; Chen, B.H. (2016). Utilization of microemulsions from Rhinacanthus nasutus (L.) kurz to improve carotenoid bioavailability. *Scientific Reports*, 6, 25426, doi: 10.1038/srep25426.

[28] Guerin, M.; Huntley, M.E.; Olaizola, M. (2003). Haematococcus astaxanthin: applications for human health and nutrition. *Trends in Biotechnology*, 21, 210-216.

[29] Carbonell-Capella, J.M.; Buniowska, M.; Barba, F.J.; Esteve, M.; Frígola, A. (2014). Analytical methods for determining bioavailability and bioaccessibility of bioactivecompounds from fruits and vegetables: a review. *Comprehensive Reviews in Food Science and Food Safety*, 13, 155-171.

[30] Mercadante, A. Z. (2008). *Food colorants – chemical and functional properties*, New York.

[31] Saini, R.K.; NILE, S.H.; PARK, S.W. (2015). Carotenoids from fruits and vegetables: chemistry, analysis, occurrence, bioavailability and biological activities. *Food Research International*, 76, 735-750.

[32] Britton, G.; Liaaen-Jensen, S.; Pfander, H. (2004). *Carotenoids: handbook*. Badel, Birkhäuser Verlag.

[33] Prasanna, R.; Sood, A.; Jaiswal, P.; Nayak, S.; Gupta, V.; Chaudhary, V.; Joshi, M.; Natarajan, C. (2010). Rediscovering cyanobacteria as valuable sources of bioactive compounds (Review). *Applied Biochemistry and Microbiology*, 46, 119-134.

[34] Walter, M. H.; Strack, D. (2011). Carotenoids and their cleavage products: biosynthesis and functions. *Natural Product Reports*, 28, 663–692.

[35] Paliwal, C.; Ghosh, T.; George, B.; Pancha, I.; Maurya, R.; Chokshi, k.; Ghosh, A.; Mishra, S. (2015). Microalgal carotenoids: potential nutraceutical compounds with chemotaxonomic importance. *Algal Research*, 15, 24-31.

[36] Goiris, k.; Muylaert, K.; Fraeye, I.; Foubert, M.; Brabanter, J.; Cooman, L. (2012) Antioxidant potential of microalgae in relation to their phenolic and carotenoid content. *Journal of Applied Phycology*, 24, 1477-1486.

[37] Chen, C.; Jesisca.; Hsieh, C.; Lee, D.; Chang, C.; Chang, J.; (2016). Production, extraction and stabilization of lutein from microalga Chlorella sorokiniana MB-1. *Bioresource Technology*, 200, 500-505.

[38] IP, P.; CHEN, F. (2005). Production of astaxanthin by the green microalga Chlorella zofingiensis in the dark. *Process Biochemistry*, 40, 733-738.

[39] Han, D.; Li, Y.; Hu, Q. (2013). Astaxanthin in microalgae: pathways, functions and biotechnological implications. *Algae*, 28, 131-147.

[40] Kim, D.; Vijayan, D.; Praveenkumar, R.; Han, J.; Lee, K.; Park, J.; Chang, W.; Lee, J.; Oh, Y. (2016). Cell-wall disruption and lipid/astaxanthin extraction from microalgae: Chlorella and Haematococcus. *Bioresource Technology*, 199, 300-310.

[41] Albrecht, M.; Takaichi, S.; Steiger, S.; Wang, Z.Y.; Sandmann, G. (2000). Novel hydroxycarotenoids with improved antioxidative properties produced by gene combination in Escherichia coli. *Nature Biotechnology*, 18, 843–846.

[42] Klassen, J.L.; Foght, J.M. (2011). Characterization of Hymenobacter isolates from Victoria upper glacier, Antarctica reveals five new species and substantial non-vertical evolution within this genus. *Extremophiles*, 15, 45-57.

[43] Rao, A.V.; Rao, L.G. (2007). Carotenoids and human health. *Pharmacological Research*, 55, 207-216.

[44] García-González, M.; Moreno, J.; Manzano, J.C.; Florencio, F.J.; Guerrero, M.G. (2005). Production of Dunaliella salina biomass rich in 9-cis-ß-carotene and lutein in a closed tubular photobioreactor. *Journal of Biotechnology*, 115, 81-90.

[45] Fernandez-Garcia E.; Carvajal-Lerida I.; Jaren-Galan M.; Garrido-Fernandez J.; Perez-Galvez A.; Hornero-Mendez D. (2012). Carotenoids bioavailability from foods: From plant pigments to efficient biological activities. *Food Research International*, 46, 438–450.

[46] Lerfall, J. (2016). Carotenoids: occurrence, properties and determination. *Encyclopedia of Food and Health*, http://dx.doi.org/10.1016/B978-0-12-384947-2.00119-7.

[47] Stahl, W.; Sies, H. (2005). Bioactivity and protective effects of natural carotenoids. *Biochimica et Biophysica Acta*, 1740, 101-107.

[48] Fiedor, J.; Burda, K. (2014). Potential role of carotenoids as antioxidants in human health and disease. *Nutrients*, 6, 466-488.

[49] Landrum, J.T. (2010). *Carotenoids: physical, chemical, and biological functions and properties*, United States.

[50] Cvetkovic, D.; Fiedor, L.; Fiedor, J.; Wisniewska-Becker, A.; Markovic, D. (2014). *Carotenoids: Food Sources, Production and Health Benefits*, New York.

[51] El-Agamey, A.; Lowe, G.M.; McGarvey, D.J.; Mortensen. A.; Phillip, D.M.; Truscott, T.G.; Young, A.J. (2004). Carotenoid radical chemistry and antioxidant/pro-oxidant properties. *Archives of Biochemistry and Biophysics*, 430, 37–48.

[52] Miki W. (1991). Biological functions and activities of animal carotenoids. *Pure and Applied Chemistry*, 63, 141-146.

[53] Gouveia, L.; Empis, J. (2003). Relative stabilities of microalgal carotenoids in microalgal extracts, biomass and fish feed: effect of storage conditions. *Innovative Food Science and Emerging Technologies*, 4, 227-233.

[54] Yamashita, E. (2013). Astaxanthin as a medical food. *Functional Foods in Health and Disease*, 3, 254-258.

[55] Reyes, F.A.; Mendiola, J.A.; Mendiola, J.A.; Suárez-Alvarez, S.; Ibañez, E.; Valle, J.M. (2016). Adsorbent-assisted supercritical CO2 extraction of carotenoids from Neochloris oleoabundans paste. *The Journal of Supercritical Fluids*, 112, 7-13.

[56] Brand, W. (2006). Flavonoid-mediated inhibition of intestinal ABC transporters may affect the oral bioavailability of drugs, food-borne toxic compounds and bioactive ingredients. *Biomedicine & Pharmacotherapy*, 60, 508–519.

[57] Werman, M.J.; Ben-Amotz, A.; Mokady, S. (1999). Availability and antiperoxidative effects of b-carotene from Dunaliella bardawil in alcohol-drinking rats. *Research Communications*, 10, 449-454.

[58] Boh, T. (2008). Bioavailability of non-provitamin A carotenoids. *Current Nutrition & Food Science*, 4, 240-258.

[59] Vallejo F.; Gil-Izquierdo A.; Perez-Vicente A.; Garcia-Viguera C. (2004). In vitro gastrointestinal digestion study of broccoli inflorescence phenolic compounds, glucosinolates, and vitamin C. *Journal of Agricultural and Food Chemistry*, 52, 135-138.

[60] Queiroz, M.I.; Hornes, M.O.; Manetti, A.G.S.; Zepka, L. Q.; Jacob-Lopes, E. (2013). Fish processing wastewater as a platform of the microalgal biorefineries. *Biosystems Engineering*, 115, 195-202.

[61] Pereira, C.G.; Meireles, A. M. (2010). Supercritical Fluid Extraction of Bioactive Compounds: Fundamentals, Applications and Economic Perspectives. *Food Bioprocess Technology*, 3, 340–372.

[62] Shah, M.M.R.; Liang Y.; Cheng J.J.; Daroch, M. (2016). Astaxanthin-Producing Green Microalga Haematococcus pluvialis: From Single Cell to High Value Commercial Products. *Frontiers in Plant Science*, 7, 531.

[63] Singh, B.B.; Shakil, N. A.; Kumar, J.; Walia, S.; Kar, J. (2015). Develment of slow release formulations of ß-carotene employing amphiphilic polymers and their release kinetics study in water and different pH conditions. *Journal of Food Science and Technology*, 52, 8068–8076.

[64] Markets and Markets (2016). *Carotenoids Market by Type (Astaxanthin, Beta-Carotene, Canthaxanthin, Lutein, Lycopene, & Zeaxanthin), Source (Synthetic and Natural), Application (Supplements, Food, Feed, and Cosmetics), & by Region - Global Trends & Forecasts to 2021.* (http://www.marketsandmarkets.com). Access on 20 June 2016.

[65] Lorenz, R., & Cysewki, G. (2004). Commercial potential for Haematococcus microalgae as a natural source of astaxanthin. *Tibtech*, 18.

[66] El baz, F.K.; Aboul-Enein, A.M.; El-Baroty, G. S.; Youssef, A.M.; Abdel-Baky, H. H. (2002). Accumulation of antioxidant vitamins in Dunaliella salina. *Online Journal of Biological Sciences*, 4, 220-223.

[67] Grudzinski, W.; Krzeminska, I.; Luchowski, R.; Nosalewicz, A.; Gruszecki, W. L. (2016). Strong-light-induced yellowing of green microalgae Chlorella: A study on molecular mechanisms of the acclimation response. *Algal Research*, 16, 245-254.

[68] Panis, G.; Carreon, J.R. (2016). Commercial astaxanthin production derived by green alga Haematococcus pluvialis: A microalgae process model and a techno-economic assessment all through production line. *Algal Research*, 18, 175-190.

[69] Chiu, P.; Soong, K.; Chen, C.N. (2016). Cultivation of two thermotolerant microalgae under tropical conditions: Influences of carbon sources and light duration on biomass and lutein productivity in four seasons. *Bioresource Technology*, 212, 190-198.

[70] Abrahamsson, I.; Rodriguez-Meizoso, C.; Turner. (2015). Supercritical fluid extraction of lipids from linseed with on-line evaporative light scattering detection, *Analytica Chimica Acta*, 853, 320-327.

[71] Gayathri, S.; Rajasree, S.R.R.; Kirubagaran, R.; Aranganathan, L.; Suman, T.Y. (2016). Spectral characterization of ß, e-carotene-3, 3'-diol

(lutein) from marine microalgae Chlorella salina. *Renewable Energy*, 98, 78-93.

[72] Jaime, L.; Rodríguez-Meizoso, I.; Cifuentes, A.; Santoyo, S.; Suarez, S.; Ibáñez, E.; Señorans, F.J. (2010). Pressurized liquids as an alternative process to antioxidante carotenoids' extraction from Haematococcus pluvialis microalgae. *LWT-Food Science and Technology*, 43, 105-112.

[73] Leya, T.; Rahn, A.; Lutz, C.; Remias, D. (2009). Response of arctic snowand permafrost algae to high light and nitrogen stress by changes in pigment compositionand applied aspects for biotechnology. *FEMS Microbiology Letters*, 67, 432-443.

[74] Hu, C.; Lin, J.; Lu, F.; Chou, F.; Yang, D. (2008). Determination of carotenoids in Dunaliella salina cultivated in Taiwan and antioxidant capacity of the algal carotenoid extract. *Food Chemistry*, 109, 439-446.

In: Carotenoids
Editors: Hanne Leif and Felix Ulrik

ISBN: 978-1-53612-685-3

Chapter 3

The Fate of Carotenoid Contents in Apple Varieties with Different Scald Susceptibility

Alexis Marsol-Vall[1], Albert Tomàs[1], Mercè Balcells[1], Francisca Vilaró[2] and Ramon Canela-Garayoa[1,*]
[1]Department of Chemistry-Agrotecnio,
University of Lleida, ETSEA, Lleida, Spain
[2]Scientific Technical Service DATCEM,
University of Lleida, ETSEA, Lleida, Spain

Abstract

A statical approach based on Principal Component Analysis (PCA) was performed to study the contents of carotenoids present in the cuticle of four apple varieties (Golden Reinders; Fuji Zhen Aztec; Fuji Fubrax and Superchief) with different scald susceptibility after harvest and low temperature storage. The scald phenomenon results from the damage and death within the surface layers of cells in localized regions of apple and pears. Our study demonstrates that the four apples varieties showed different carotenoid profiles in the cuticle and also that the fate of these carotenoids was different during the conservation of the four varieties at low temperature for 7 month. The two PCs explained 81.4% of the

* Corresponding Author Email: canela@quimica.udl.cat.

variability at harvest. A clear separation in PC1 between the two Fuji cultivars and Golden Reinders and Superchief was observed. In addition, the loadings plot indicated that Fuji cultivars had a more heterogeneous content of carotenoids, while Superchief and Golden Reinders were highly correlated with β-carotene, (all-*E*)-lutein and (all-*E*)-violaxanthin. In contrast, more biosynthetic evolved oxidized carotenoids, such as luteoxanthin isomers, neochrome and neoxhanthin isomers, would explain the behaviour of the Fuji varieties. After seven months of cold storage PC1 and PC2 explained 86.4% of the variability of carotenoid. A clear separation of the four cultivars was observed. In this regard, as in samples at harvest, the scores plot revealed separation between Fuji cultivars and Golden Reinders, and Superchief in the PC1. However, in this case, a separation between Golden Reinders and Superchief is shown in PC2. The loadings plot indicates that Fuji cultivars presented a higher correlation with diverse carotenoids, mainly those same oxocarotenoids as at the time of harvesting. Superchief was still positively correlated with the content of (all-*E*)-lutein. (9'Z)-Neoxanthin also appeared to be responsible for the PC1 differentiation between Golden Reinders and Superchief, and the two Fuji varieties. In addition, neochrome and auroxanthin B, and β-carotene would participate in the PC2 differentiation between Golden Reinders and Superchief. We hypothesize that the different scald susceptibility of the four apples varieties could partially be a consequence of these differences in profile and fate. Indeed, carotenoids are considered natural antioxidants, however their antioxidant capability depends on their chemical structure.

1. INTRODUCTION

Superficial scald is a physiological disorder that affects fruits such as apple and pear. It is characterized by tissue damage on the fruit surface, resulting in reduced quality [1]. Apples (Malus domestica Borkh.) are generally stored at low temperature for long periods, during which they show symptoms of scald development very similar to those produced by chilling injury [2]. Many factors, including cultivar variety (specific apple varieties such as 'Granny Smith', 'Red Delicious', 'Pink Lady' and 'Fuji' are more susceptible to the onset of this disorder than others such as 'Golden Delicious'), maturity, seasonal environmental variation, cultural practices, postharvest storage conditions, and certain treatments have been reported to affect scald development [1-5]. Although the specific mechanism underlying scald is unknown, it is believed that the biosynthesis of α-farnesene and its subsequent degradation to conjugated trienes cause the disruption, discoloration, and death of surface cells [6-8]. However, other studies have reported that oxidation products of α-farnesene are not essential for scald development in fruit with severely compromised anti-oxidative defences. Nevertheless, free radicals and/or toxic volatiles generated by α-farnesene oxidation can lead to an increase in the expression and intensity of scald symptoms [9]. Also, it has been described that α-farnesene levels are very low in the skin of apples at harvest and that α-farnesene content and α-farnesene synthase activity increase rapidly during fruit storage at 0°C [10].

Given the occurrence of superficial scald on apples during long storage, several approaches to prevent this injury, including storage under a controlled low oxygen atmosphere, forced ventilation, and 1-methylcyclopropene (1-MCP) treatment, have been implemented [11]. However, their efficacy is strongly determined by the maturity stage and uniformity of the fruit batch [9, 12, 13]. Recent years have witnessed the emergence of techniques that use natural compounds with anti-oxidative capacity to prevent or reduce superficial scald. In this regard, the reduction of polyphenol content in apple peel via polymerization is accompanied by an increase in superficial scald [14-16]. In addition to the effect of polyphenols on scald control, other authors have proposed that lipophilic compounds present in apple skin participate in scald control [17]. Indeed, highly lipophilic carotenoids, a group of natural anti-oxidants, are present in apple peel. Carotenoids are natural pigments that serve a multitude of functions. They are synthesized by a huge range of organisms within archaea and eubacteria (including cyanobacteria), as well as eukaryotes (algae, fungi and plants). They are found in a large number of fruits and vegetables (oranges, tomatoes, carrots, spinach, sweet potatoes, and pumpkins), spices (paprika), some animal products (eggs, butter, milk) and seafood (salmon, shrimp, trout, mollusk, etc.). Carotenoids are required for the correct assembly of photosystems in plants. These pigments absorb light across a broader range of the spectral region in which the sun irradiates maximally and they transfer the energy to chlorophyll, thereby initiating the photochemical events of photosynthesis. In addition, carotenoids serve as precursors for the hormones abscisic acid (ABA) and strigolactones. They also act as attractants for animals, such as pollinating insects and seed-disbursing herbivores. Carotenoids also have a number of functions in animals. For example, they boost the immune system and promote general health. These pigments are critical in determining sexual behavior and reproduction processes. They also help to prevent predation and parasitism. In humans, carotenoids are precursors of vitamin A, this being one of their most important physiological functions. These pigments are also known to contribute to the prevention of and protection against serious health disorders such as cancer, heart disease, and macular degeneration. Carotenoids are used in industry: (a) in nutrient supplementation; (b) for pharmaceutical purposes; (c) in animal feed; (d) as food colorants (such as bixin and crocetin, found in annatto seeds and saffron respectively); and (e) in fragrances (such as ionones, damascones, and damascenones). Consequently, these pigments have been extensively studied by organic and food chemists, biologists, physiologists, medical doctors, and recently also by environmental scientists. The widespread interest in carotenoids has led to an increased demand for reliable analytical methodologies [18]. However, the relationship between individual carotenoids and scald susceptibility has not been addressed to date [19].

Solid–liquid extraction is the most widely used technique to analyse carotenoids in solid vegetable matrices [20]. These compounds generally differ in solubility properties, thus the choice of extraction solvent and the use of a saponification step will greatly affect carotenoid extraction. Various solvents have been used for this purpose, depending on the sample and the sort of compounds expected in the sample [21]. Once carotenoids have been extracted, reversed-phase high-performance liquid chromatography (HPLC), mainly with C30 stationary phases [22, 23] and C18 stationary phases, have been used to determine their profile and content [16, 24]. Commercial standards, when available, are used for identification purposes. However, as many carotenoid standards are not commercially available, ultraviolet–visible (UV–vis), mass spectra and published information on retention times are also useful for this purpose.

Here we compared the carotenoid profile in four apple cultivars (Golden Reinders; Fuji Zhen Aztec; Fuji Fubrax and Superchief) that differ in susceptibility to scald. This profile was studied at harvest and seven months after storage at 1.5°C and 94% of relative humidity in an ultra-low oxygen (ULO) atmosphere. Finally, Principal Component Analysis (PCA) was used to determine the influence of lipidic anti-oxidants in the mechanism underlying the scald process.

2. Materials and Methods

2.1. Reagents, Solvents and Carotenoid Standards

Methanol, 2-propanol, hexane, diethyl ether, acetonitrile (ACN) and acetone (HPLC grade purity) were supplied by J.T. Baker (Deventer, The

Netherlands). The chromatographic solvents were ACN, methanol (LC–MS grade), also from J.T. Baker, and water was purified in a Milli-Q system from Millipore (Bedford, MA, USA). Sodium chloride was provided by Fluka (Buchs SG, Switzerland) and potassium hydroxide by Panreac (Barcelona, Spain). Diethyl ether was stored under an argon atmosphere at 4°C to prevent the formation of peroxides.

β-Carotene, (all-*E*)-lutein and β-cryptoxanthin were purchased from Sigma–Aldrich Fine Chemicals (Madrid, Spain). (all-*E*)-Zeaxanthin was supplied by Fluka. Phytoene, (all-*E*)-violaxanthin, (9′*Z*)-neoxanthin and (all-*E*)-antheraxanthin were supplied by CaroteNature (Lupsingen, Switzerland).

All stock standard solutions were prepared in ACN:MeOH:acetone (47:20:33, v/v/v) and stored at −80°C.

2.2. Samples

Samples of apple cultivars with different susceptibility to superficial scald were supplied by Nufri (Mollerussa, Spain). The following cultivars were examined: Golden Reinders (GR); Fuji Zhen Aztec (FZ); Fuji Fubrax (FF): and Superchief (SC). The first cultivar shows low susceptibility to superficial scald, followed by the two Fuji cultivars. Finally, SC is known to be highly susceptible to this skin injury. Samples were supplied at harvest and after seven months of cold storage at 1.5°C and 94% of relative humidity in an ultra-low oxygen (ULO) atmosphere.

Samples were processed upon receipt. Each sample comprised ten apples, which were cut into four sections and peeled. Peel was placed on a filter paper and immediately frozen with liquid nitrogen prior to being freeze-dried at −50°C, 1.1 Pa for 24 h in a Cryodos −50 lyophilizer (Telstar, Terrassa, Spain).

2.3. Extraction Procedure

Aliquots between 0.5 and 1 g of lyophilized and ground apple peel were weighed in a 15-mL Falcon tube. Then, 3 mL of methanol was added, and the mixture was shaken for 10 min. Next, 6 mL of chloroform was added, and the mixture shaken (10 min). Afterwards, 2.3 mL of a solution of 10% NaCl (w/v) was added. The mixture was shaken for 15 min and cooled at 4°C. The mixture was centrifuged at 2700 x *g* for 3 min at 4ºC, and the organic layer was recovered. The aqueous phase was re-extracted with 2 mL of hexane:diethyl ether (3:1, v/v) for 10 min and centrifuged under the same conditions. The organic solutions were combined in a 5-mL glass tube and dried under a nitrogen stream at room temperature.

The dry residue was saponified in a shaking incubator (211DS; Labnet, Edison, NJ, USA) for 60 min at 55°C under N_2 using 1 mL of a solution of 6% KOH in methanol (w/v). After the addition of 1 mL of a solution of 10% NaCl (w/v), the mixture was kept in a freezer for 15 min. Then, 2.5 mL of hexane:diethyl ether (3:1, v/v) was added, and the mixture was vortexed and centrifuged at 433 × *g* for 3 min (this step was repeated until the aqueous phase was colourless). The organic layers were combined, and the solvent was removed under nitrogen stream. The residue was stored at −80°C under nitrogen until UPLC analysis. The dry residue was dissolved in the injection solvent immediately prior to analysis.

2.4. Ultra-Performance Liquid Chromatography

Chromatographic analysis was performed on a Waters ACQUITY UPLC™ system (Waters, Milford, MA, USA) consisting of an ACQUITY UPLC™ binary solvent manager and ACQUITY UPLC™ sample manager, coupled to a photodiode array (PDA) 2996 detector. Compounds were separated using an ACQUITY UPLC™ BEH C18 column (1.7 µm; 2.1 mm × 150 mm) (Waters, Manchester, UK) and a gradient system with the mobile phase consisting of solvent A, ACN–MeOH (7:3, v/v) and solvent B, 100% H_2O. The linear gradient was as follows: 0–1.03 min, 25% B, 0.5 mL/min (isocratic); 1.03–9.88 min, 4.9% B 0.5 mL/min (linear gradient); 9.88–11.38 min, 0% B, 0.7 mL/min (linear gradient); 11.38–20.18 min, 0% B, 0.7 mL/min (isocratic); 20.18–21.00 min, 25% B, 0.5 mL/min (linear gradient); and 21.00–23.00 min, 25% B, 0.5 mL/min (isocratic). The weak and strong needle solvents were ACN–MeOH (7:3, v/v) and 2-propanol, respectively. The injection volume was 5 µL and the column was kept at 32ºC and the injector at 25ºC. A wavelength of λ=450 nm was used for quantification. Instrumental control, data acquisition, and processing were carried out using MassLynx™ software (version 4.1; Waters, USA).

2.5. Mass Spectrometry

MS analysis was carried out on a Waters ACQUITY TQD tandem quadrupole mass spectrometer (Waters, UK). The instrument was operated using an atmospheric pressure chemical ionization (APCI) source in positive ion mode. The APCI parameters were as follows: corona voltage 4.0 kV; extractor voltage 3 V; source temperature 150°C; probe temperature 450°C; desolvation temperature 150°C; cone gas (nitrogen) flow 10 L/h; and desolvation gas (also nitrogen) flow 150 L/h. Collision-induced dissociation was achieved using argon as the collision gas at a flow rate of 0.12 mL/min in the collision cell. Data acquisition was performed using MassLynx 4.1 software (Waters, USA).

2.6. Data Analysis

Principal Component Analysis (PCA) was performed with the Unscrambler 9.7 software (CAMO Software AS, Oslo, Norway). All compounds included in the PCA were previously normalized according to the standard deviation of the samples, in order to standardize the values and give an equal weight in the model. PCA is an unsupervised technique that reduces the dimensionality of the data set but retains the maximum amount of variability [25].

3. Results and Discussion

3.1. Carotenoid Profiling

Identification of carotenoids with the corresponding analytical standard was limited because many of them are not commercially available. Therefore, identification was based on commercial standards and on results previously published on fruit juice samples [26]. The usefulness of published data on C18 [24] phases, together with the UV–vis absorption spectra (namely, the wavelength of the absorption maxima and the spectral fine structure), to identify carotenoids has already been reported. Moreover, it is widely known that some carotenoids have a very similar chemical composition and structure, thus MS using APCI in positive ionization mode confirms carotenoid identification by providing the molecular weight and fragmentation patterns [27].

Table 1 reports on the main carotenoids identified in the apple peel samples, and Figure 1 shows a typical chromatogram for an apple sample (peaks are numbered as in Table 1).

Table 1. Retention time and UV-Vis parameters for compounds found in apple peel samples

Compound n.	Compound name	Retention time	λmax (nm)
1	(all-*E*)-Neoxanthin [b]	4.96	418;442;471
2	Neochrome [b]	5.08	400;423;451
3	(9'*Z*)-Neoxanthin [a]	5.62	329;414;438;466
4	(all-*E*)-Violaxanthin [a]	5.78	417;442;471
5	(all-*E*)-LuteoxanthinA [b, c]	6.89	401;424;450
6	(all-*E*)-LuteoxanthinB [b, c]	7.17	401;424;450
7	(all-*E*)-Antheraxanthin [a]	7.40	422;448;475
8	AuroxanthinA [b, c]	7.53	384;403;428
9	AuroxanthinB [b, c]	7.84	384;403;428
10	(9'*Z*)-LuteoxanthinA [b, c]	8.21	313;396;418;445
11	(9'*Z*)-Violaxanthin [b]	8.36	328;414;437;466
12	(9'*Z*)-LuteoxanthinB [b, c]	8.44	313;396;418;445
13	(all-*E*)-Zeaxanthin [a]	8.63	428;453;478
14	(all-*E*)-Lutein [a]	8.79	424;447;475
15	Lutein isomer [b]	9.65	332;419;449;471
16	β-Cryptoxanthin [a]	12.58	424;452;479
17	β-Carotene [a]	16.33	422;452;479

[a] Identification performed on the basis of the UV–vis spectrum and specific mass fragments of the standard compounds.

[b] Tentative identification on the basis of UV–vis spectrum, MS, fine structure, HPLC/UPLC retention times, and published data.

[c] The assignation of the configuration of the 8 or 8′ carbon in these peaks was not possible using UV–vis absorption and MS spectra. Therefore they were named A and B.

Table 2 shows an increase in overall carotenoid content for all the varieties examined after seven months of storage at low temperature. This effect is related with the maturation process of the fruits during storage, which is highly related with a decrease in the content of chlorophylls.

Table 2. Estimate carotenoid content (μg/g) for the four cultivars measured at 450 nm at harvest and after seven months of cold storage

Compound	Golden Reinders		Fuji Zhen Aztec		Fuji Fubrax		Superchief	
	At harvest	After storage	At harvest	After storage	At harvest	After storage	At harvest	After storage
(all-*E*)-Neoxanthin	0.18	2.13	0.31	5.34	n.d.	5.44	n.d.	1.31
Neochrome	1.32	1.44	1.55	0.78	1.83	0.78	0.64	0.45
(9'Z)-Neoxanthin	0.88	1.05	0.87	0.78	0.99	0.73	0.50	1.24
(all-*E*)-Violaxanthin	0.57	0.92	0.38	5.63	0.30	5.63	0.58	1.60
(all-*E*)-LuteoxanthinA	0.53	0.86	1.15	0.89	0.77	0.78	n.d.	0.64
(all-*E*)-LuteoxanthinB	0.81	1.28	1.72	1.42	1.16	1.27	0.19	1.03
(all-*E*)-Antheraxanthin	n.d.	0.10	0.09	0.64	n.d.	0.56	n.d.	0.10
AuroxanthinA	n.d.	n.d.	0.16	n.d.	0.19	n.d.	n.d.	0.19
AuroxanthinB	n.d.	0.14	0.10	0.10	n.d.	0.13	n.d.	0.08
(9'Z)-LuteoxanthinA	1.08	1.18	2.91	1.71	2.99	1.95	n.d.	0.81
(9'Z)-Violaxanthin	0.84	2.45	1.61	11.66	0.79	12.49	n.d.	2.66
(9'Z)-LuteoxanthinB	0.82	0.94	1.88	1.35	1.89	1.45	0.38	0.66
(all-*E*)-Zeaxanthin	0.19	0.18	0.55	0.61	0.51	0.44	n.d.	0.12
(all-*E*)-Lutein	2.34	5.34	1.39	5.23	1.19	4.73	5.10	6.61
β-Cryptoxanthin	n.d.	0.18	n.d.	0.76	n.d.	0.72	n.d.	0.14
β-Carotene	0.15	0.79	0.36	1.29	0.24	1.07	0.54	1.00
Total carotenoids	**9.70**	**19.06**	**15.24**	**38.81**	**13.09**	**38.74**	**7.92**	**18.69**

n.d.: not detected.

This phenomenon has been usually linked to an over regulation of the genetic expression of carotenes (phytoene synthase) [28]. This enzyme catalyses the formation of phytoene, which is a precursor in the carotenoids synthetic pathway. Considering each of the cultivars, it can be observed that the carotenoids that show a higher increase are (all-*E*)-neoxanthin, (all-*E*)-lutein, (9'*Z*)-violaxanthin and β-carotene in Golden Reinders; (all-*E*)-neoxanthin, (all-*E*)-violaxanthin, (9'*Z*)-violaxanthin, (all-*E*)-lutein, β-carotene in Fuji Zhen Aztec and Fuji Fubrax; and (all-*E*)-neoxanthin, (all-*E*)-violaxanthin, (9'*Z*)-luteoxanthinA and (all-*E*)-luteoxanthinB in Superchief.

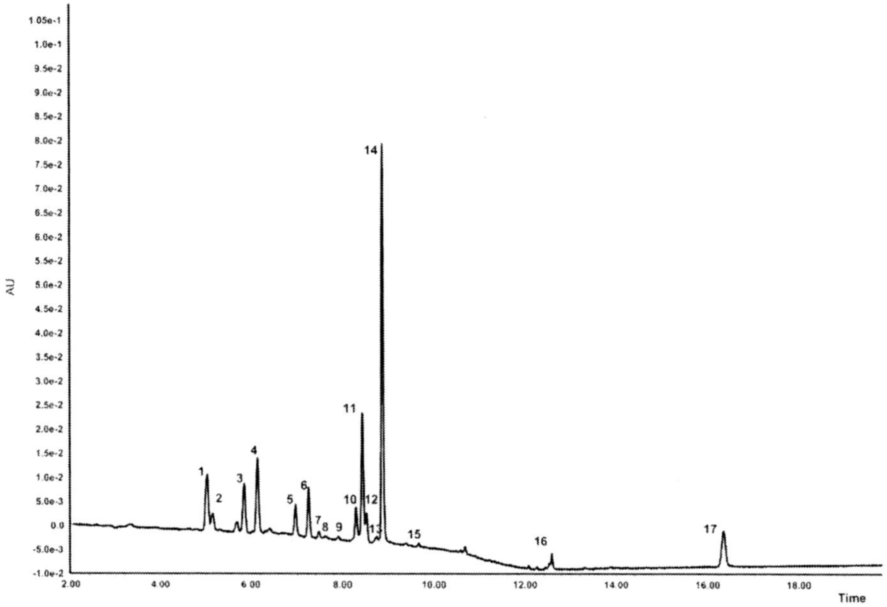

Figure 1. UPLC carotenoid profile at λ= 450 nm of Golden Reinders apple peel sample (carotenoids numbered as in Table 1).

3.2. Carotenoid Distribution at Harvest

To correlate the individual carotenoid content and apple cultivars with susceptibility to superficial scald, we performed a PCA analysis. The two PCs explained 81.4% of the variability. Figure 2a shows a clear separation in PC1 between the two Fuji cultivars and Golden Reinders and Superchief. In addition, the loadings plot (Figure 2b) indicates that Fuji cultivars have a more heterogeneous content of carotenoids, while Superchief and Golden Reinders are highly correlated with β-carotene (17), (all-*E*)-lutein (14) and (all-*E*)-violaxanthin (4). The putative lutein isomer (15) also participates in the PC1 differentiation between Fuji cultivars and the two other cultivars. In contrast, more biosynthetic evolved oxidized carotenoids, such as luteoxanthins (6, 10, and 11), neochrome (2) and neoxhanthins (1 and 3), would explain the behaviour of the Fuji varieties [29].

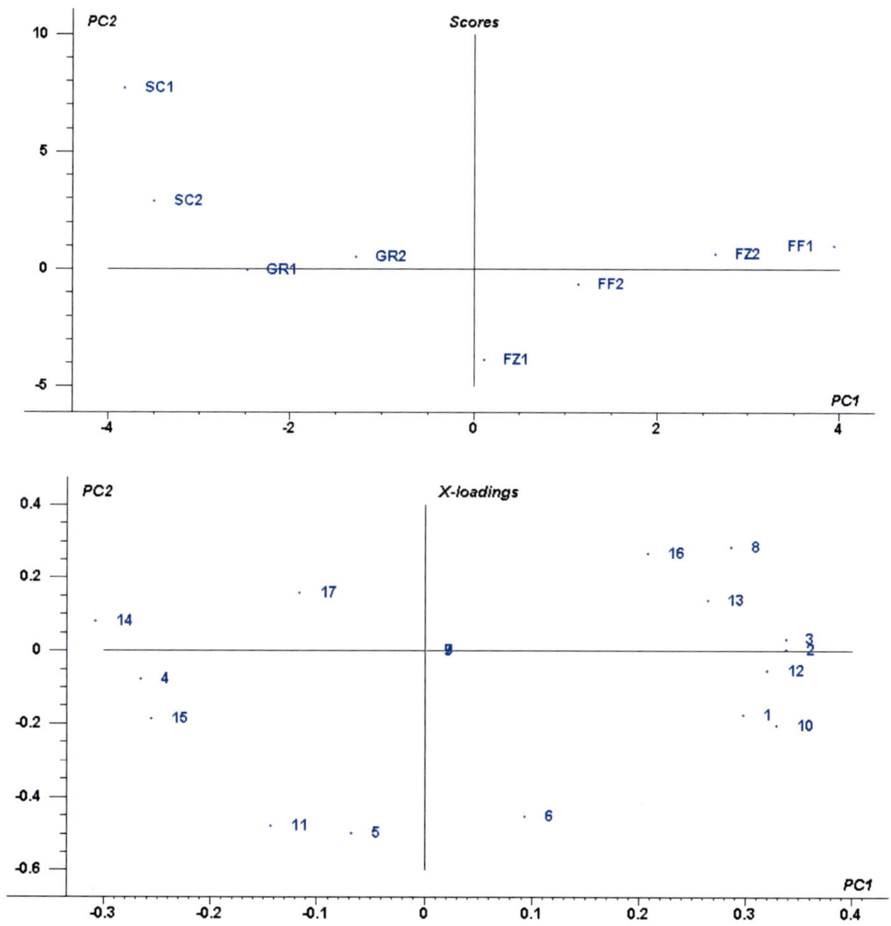

Figure 2. PCA plot of the four apple cultivars at harvest. A) Scores plot. B) Loadings plot.

3.3. Carotenoid Distribution after Seven Months of Cold Storage

In the PCA analysis, PC1 and PC2 explained 86.4% of the variability of carotenoid distribution after seven months of cold storage. Figure 3a shows a clear separation of the four cultivars. In this regard, as in samples at harvest, the scores plot revealed separation between Fuji cultivars and Golden Reinders, and Superchief in the PC1. However, in this case, a separation between Golden Reinders and Superchief is shown in PC2.

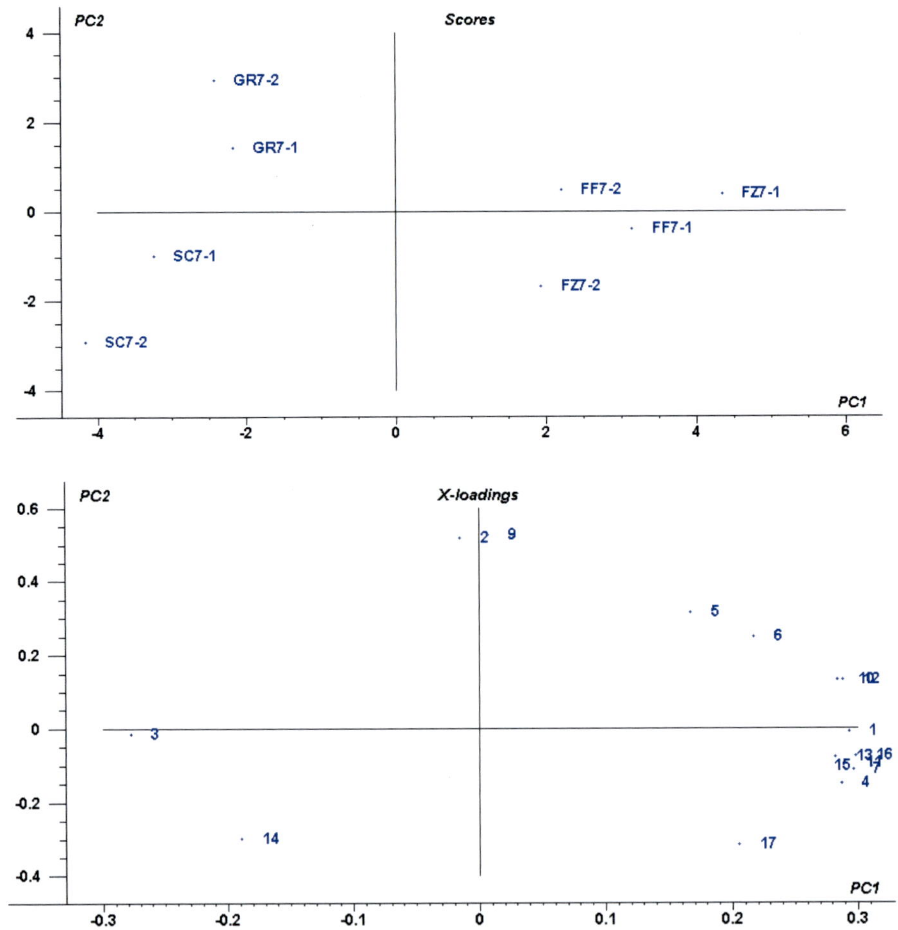

Figure 3. PCA plot of the four apple cultivars after seven months of cold storage. A) Scores plot. B) Loadings plot.

The loadings plot indicates that Fuji cultivars present a higher correlation with diverse carotenoids, mainly those same oxocarotenoids as at the time of harvesting. Superchief is still positively correlated with the content of (all-*E*)-lutein (14). (9'*Z*)-Neoxanthin (3) also appears to be responsible for the PC1 differentiation between Golden Reinders and Superchief, and the two Fuji varieties. In addition, neochrome (2) and auroxanthin B (9), and β-carotene (17) would participate in the PC2 differentiation between Golden Reinders and Superchief.

The relative decrease in lutein, β-carotene and, to a less extent, violaxanthin (4) in Golden Reinders versus Superchief, together with the relative increase in neochrome (2) and auroxanthin B (9) in Golden Reinders, could explain the higher anti-oxidant capacity of the former variety. In fact, lutein is present at the end of the metabolic carotenoid pathway, which starts from α-carotene, whereas neochrome and auroxanthin are at the end of the metabolic transformation of violaxanthin, a carotenoid derived from the oxidation of β-carotene. Neoxanthin also derives from violaxanthin and it is the precursor of neochrome [30]. This different degree of oxidation in the carotenoids could explain the higher susceptibility of Superchief than Golden Reinders to scald. Indeed, the transformation of carotenes to highly oxidized carotenoids seems to be far less relevant in Superchief than in Golden Reinders. The intermediate susceptibility of the two Fuji varieties could be related to the presence of high contents of epoxicarotenoids, such as the various luteoxanthin isomers and violaxanthin, even at harvesting.

ACKNOWLEDGMENTS

This work was supported in part by a Grant-in-Aid from the Departament d'Universitats, Recerca i Societat de la Informació of the Generalitat de Catalunya (2014 SGR 1296 Agricultural Biotechnology Research Group). The authors would like to thank the company NUFRI (Mollerussa, Spain) for supplying the samples used in this study.

REFERENCES

[1] Emongor, V., Murr, D., Lougheed, E. (1994). Preharvest factors that predispose apples to superficial scald. *Postharvest Biology and Technology,* 4: 289-300.

[2] Watkins, C. B., Bramlage, W. J., Brookfield, P. L., Reid, S. J., Weis, S. A., Alwan, T. F. (2000). Cultivar and growing region influence efficacy of warming treatments for amelioration of superficial scald development on apples after storage. *Postharvest Biology and Technology*, 19: 33-45.

[3] Ferguson, I., Volz, R., Woolf, A. (1999). Preharvest factors affecting physiological disorders of fruit. *Postharvest Biology and Technology,* 15: 255-262.

[4] Ingle, M., D'souza, M. (1989). Physiology and control of superficial scald of apples: a review. *HortScience* (USA), 24:28–31.

[5] Tsantili, E., Gapper, N. E., Arquiza, J. A., Whitaker, B. D., Watkins, C. B. (2007). Ethylene and α-farnesene metabolism in green and red skin of three apple cultivars in response to 1-methylcyclopropene (1-MCP) treatment. *Journal of Agricultural and Food Chemistry,* 55: 5267-5276.

[6] Anet, E. F. (1974). Superficial scald, a functional disorder of stored apples. XI. Apple antioxidants. *Journal of the Science of Food and Agriculture*, 25: 299-304.

[7] Bramlage, W., Barden, C., Watkins, C. (1993). Comparing potential predictors of scald susceptibility of apples (Malus domestica Borkh.). *Acta Horticulturae*, 326: 237-244.

[8] Eisenstecken, D., Stürz, S., Robatscher, P., Huck, C. W., Zanella, A., Oberhuber, M. (2016). Near-infrared reflection spectroscopy and partial least squares regression to predict α-farnesene and conjugated trienol content in apples during storage. *Postharvest Biology and Technology*, 117: 49-56.

[9] Whitaker, B. D., Nock, J. F., Watkins, C. B. (2000). Peel tissue α-farnesene and conjugated trienol concentrations during storage of 'White Angel'×'Rome Beauty'hybrid apple selections susceptible and resistant to superficial scald. *Postharvest Biology and Technology,* 20: 231-241.

[10] Rupasinghe, H., Paliyath, G., Murr, D. (1998). Biosynthesis of α-Farnesene and its Relation to Superficial Scald Development inDelicious' Apples. *Journal of the American Society for Horticultural Science,* 123: 882-886.

[11] Lurie, S., Watkins, C. B. (2012). Superficial scald, its etiology and control. *Postharvest Biology and Technology,* 65: 44-60.

[12] Wilkinson, B., Fidler, J. (1973). Injuries to the skin of the fruit. *The Biology of Apple and Pear Storage,* 67-80.

[13] Wang, Z., Dilley, D. R. (1999). Control of superficial scald of apples by low-oxygen atmospheres. *HortScience,* 34: 1145-1151.

[14] Piretti, M. V., Gallerani, G. Pratella, G. C. (1994). Polyphenol fate and superficial scald in apple. *Postharvest Biology and Technology,* 4: 213-224.

[15] Ju, Z., Yuan, Y., Liu, C., Zhan, S., Wang, M. (1996). Relationships among simple phenol, flavonoid and anthocyanin in apple fruit peel at harvest and scald susceptibility. *Postharvest Biology and Technology*, 8: 83-93.

[16] Boss, P. K., Gardner, R. C., Janssen, B. J., Ross, G. S. (1995). An apple polyphenol oxidase cDNA is up-regulated in wounded tissues. *Plant Molecular Biology*, 27: 429-433.

[17] Piretti, M., Gallerani, G., Pratella, G. (1994). Polyphenol fate and superficial scald in apple. *Postharvest Biology and Technology,* 4: 213-224.

[18] Rivera, S., Christou, P., Canela-Garayoa, R. (2014). Identification of carotenoids using mass spectrometry in positive ion mode. *Mass Spectrometry Reviews,* 33: 353-372.

[19] Leisso, R., Buchanan, D., Lee, J., Mattheis, J., Rudell, D. (2013). Cell wall, cell membrane, and volatile metabolism are altered by antioxidant treatment, temperature shifts, and peel necrosis during apple fruit storage. *Journal of Agricultural and Food Chemistry,* 61: 1373-1387.

[20] Dias, M. G., Oliveira, L., Camões, M. F. G. F. C., Nunes, B., Versloot, P., Hulshof, P. J. M. (2010). Critical assessment of three high performance liquid chromatography analytical methods for food carotenoid quantification. *Journal of Chromatography A,* 1217: 3494-3502.

[21] Taungbodhitham, A. K., Jones, G. P., Wahlqvist, M. L., Briggs, D. R. (1998). Evaluation of extraction method for the analysis of carotenoids in fruits and vegetables. *Food Chemistry,* 63: 577-584.

[22] Assunção, R. B., Mercadante, A. Z. (2003). Carotenoids and ascorbic acid composition from commercial products of cashew apple (Anacardium occidentale L.). *Journal of Food Composition and Analysis,* 16: 647-657.

[23] Kurz, C., Carle, R., Schieber, A. (2008). HPLC-DAD-MSn characterisation of carotenoids from apricots and pumpkins for the evaluation of fruit product authenticity. *Food Chemistry,* 110: 522-530.

[24] Dias, M. G., Camões, M. F. G. F. C., Oliveira, L. (2009). Carotenoids in traditional Portuguese fruits and vegetables. *Food Chemistry,* 113: 808-815.

[25] Jolliffe, I. Principal component analysis, *Wiley Online Library*, 2002.

[26] Delpino-Rius, A., Eras, J., Marsol-Vall, A., Vilaró, F., Balcells, M., Canela-Garayoa, R. (2014). Ultra performance liquid chromatography analysis to study the changes in the carotenoid profile of commercial monovarietal fruit juices. *Journal of Chromatography A,* 1331: 90-99.

[27] Rivera, S., Vilaró, F., Canela, R. (2011). Determination of carotenoids by liquid chromatography/mass spectrometry: effect of several dopants. *Analytical and Bioanalytical Chemistry*, 400: 1339-1346.

[28] Shewmaker, C. K., Sheehy, J. A., Daley, M., Colburn, S., Ke, D.Y. (1999). Seed-specific overexpression of phytoene synthase: increase in carotenoids and other metabolic effects. *The Plant Journal*, 20: 401-412.

[29] Mikami, K., Hosokawa, M. (2013) Biosynthetic pathway and health benefits of fucoxanthin, an algae-specific xanthophyll in brown seaweeds. *International Journal of Molecular sciences,* 14: 13763-13781.

[30] Asai, A., Terasaki, M., Nagao, A. (2004). An epoxide–furanoid rearrangement of spinach neoxanthin occurs in the gastrointestinal tract of mice and in vitro: Formation and cytostatic activity of neochrome stereoisomers. *The Journal of Nutrition,* 134: 2237-2243.

BIOGRAPHICAL SKETCH

Ramon Canela-Garayoa

Affiliation: Universitat de Lleida-Spain

Education: PhD in Chemistry

Research and Professional Experience: Green Chemistry

Publications Last Three Years:

Alexis Marsol-Vall, Mercè Balcells, Jordi Eras, Ramon Canela-Garayoa. A rapid gas chromatographic injection-port derivatization method for the tandem mass spectrometric determination of patulin and 5-hydroxymethylfurfural in fruit juices. *Journal of Chromatography A* 2016, 1453, 99-104.

Rubén Torregrosa, Edinson Yara-Varón, Mercè Balcells, Mercè Torres, Ramon Canela-Garayoa. Entirely solvent-free biocatalytic synthesis of solketal fatty esters from soybean seeds. *Comptes Rendus Chimie*, 2016, 19, 749–753.

E. Yara-Varón, A. S. Fabiano-Tixier, M. Balcells, R. Canela-Garayoa, Antoine Bilyc and F. Chemat. Is it possible to substitute hexane with green solvents for extraction of carotenoids? A theoretical versus experimental solubility study. *RSC Advances* 2016, 6, 27750-27759.

Marta M. Dolcet, Mercè Torres and Ramon Canela. Effect of fungal mycelia on the HPLC–UV and UV–vis spectrophotometric assessment of mycelium-bound epoxide hydrolase using glycidyl phenyl ether. *New Biotechnology*, 2016, 33, 449-459.

Novo, O., Balcells, M., Canela-Garayoa, R., Eras, J. Combining a flow reactor with spray dryer to allow the preparation of food-grade quality sodium 2-polyhydroxyalkyl-1,3-thiazolidine-4-carboxylates with a low environmental impact. *RSC Advances* 2016, 6, 6651-6557.

Alexis Marsol-Vall, Mercè Balcells, Jordi Eras, Ramon Canela-Garayoa. Injection-port derivatization coupled to GC–MS/MS for the analysis of glycosylated and non-glycosylated polyphenols in fruit samples. *Food Chem.* 2016, 204, 210–217.

Marsol-Vall, A.; Balcells, M.; Eras, J. and Canela-Garayoa, R. Comprehensive Two-dimensional Gas Chromatography Time-of-flight Mass Spectrometry to Assess the Presence of alfa, alfa-Trehalose and Other Disaccharides in Apple and Peach. *Phytochemical Analysis*, 2015, 26,279–286. DOI: 10.1002/pca.2561.

Delpino-Rius, A.; Eras, J.; Vilaró, F.; Cubero, MA.; Balcells, M.; Canela-Garayoa, R. Characterization of phenolic compounds in processed fibers from the juice industry. *Food Chem.*, 2015, 172, 575-584

Solarte, C., Balcells, M., Torres, M., Sala, N., Canela-Garayoa, R. Preparation of chiral glycerol derivatives using chemoenzymatic approaches. *RSC Advances* 2014, 4, 34623-34631.

Yara-Varón, E., Eras, J., Torres, M., Villorbina, G., Espart, A., Canela-Garayoa, R. Entrapment in polymeric material of resting cells of Aspergillus flavus with lipase activity. Application to the synthesis of ethyl laurate. *RSC Advances* 2014, 4, 38418-38424.

Torregrosa R; Balcells M; Torres M; Canela-Garayoa R. Chemoenzymatic solvent-free synthesis of 1-monopalmitin using a microwave reactor. *Natural Product Communications* 2014, 9, 1095 – 1098.

Solarte, C.; Yara-Varón, E.; Eras, J.; Torres, M.; Balcells, M.; Canela-Garayoa, R. Lipase activity and enantioselectivity of whole cells from a wild-type Aspergillius flavus strain. *J. Mol. Catal. B: Enzymatic* 2014, 100, 78-83.

Delpino-Rius, A.; Eras, J.; Marsol-Vall, A.; Vilaró, F.; Balcells, M.; Canela-Garayoa, R. Ultra-performance liquid chromatography analysis to study the changes in the carotenoid profile of commercial monovarietal fruit juices. *J. Chromatogr. A*, 2014, 1331, 90-99.

Marsol-Vall, A.; Delpino-Rius, A.; Eras, J.; Balcells, M.; Canela-Garayoa. A Fast and Reliable UHPLC-PDA Method for Determination of Patulin in Apple Food Products Using QuEChERS Extraction. *R. Food Anal. Method.*, 2014, 7, 465-471.

Breitenbach, J.; Bai, C.; Rivera, SM.; Canela, R.; Capell, T.; Christou, P.; Zhu, C.; Sandmann, G. A novel carotenoid, 4-keto-alpha-carotene, as an unexpected by-product during genetic engineering of carotenogenesis in rice callus. *Phytochemistry*, 2014, 98, 85-91.

Bai, C.; Rivera, SM.; Medina,V.; Alves, R.; Vilaprinyo, E.; Sorribas, A.; Canela, R.; Capell, T.; Sandmann, G.; Christou, P.; Zhu, C. An in vitro system for the rapid functional characterization of 20 genes involved in carotenoid biosynthesis and accumulation. *Plant J.,* 2014, 77, 464-475

Rivera, SM.; Christou, P.; Canela-Garayoa, R. Identification of carotenoids using mass spectrometry. *Mass Spectr. Rev.*, 2014, 33(5), 353-372.

Ramon Canela-Garayoa received a BS degree in Chemistry and a PhD in organic chemistry from the Autonomous University of Barcelona, Spain in 1980. He worked as scientist at UQUIFA SAE, a chemical company in Lliça de Vall Spain. He was a postdoctoral fellow at Cornell University, USA from 1982-1983. Currently, he is a Research Professor at the University of Lleida and he heads the green agrochemistry group. His current research interests include the development and application of instrumental methods for chemical analysis and the synthesis of compounds of commercial importance using renewable materials and chemo-enzymatic approaches.

In: Carotenoids
Editors: Hanne Leif and Felix Ulrik
ISBN: 978-1-53612-685-3

Chapter 4

THE COSMETIC USE OF CAROTENOIDS

Joanna Igielska-Kalwat*
Faculty of Chemistry,
Laboratory of Applied Adam Mickiewicz University, Poznan, Poland

ABSTRACT

According to recent canons of beauty, the skin touched by the sun signifies healthy lifestyle and wellbeing. The skin makes an excellent model to study the process of ageing. It is directly exposed to destructive effect of the elements and hence more prone to ageing than other organs of the body. Ageing is a multifactorial process controlled by both genetic and environmental factors. Carotenoids, which belong to the best known natural antioxidants, have been for many years the subject of studies aimed at their possible application in cosmetic industry. Carotenoids contain 11 coupled double bonds, so they can be classified as polyisoprenoids and they are weakly polar. Provitamin A assists in regeneration of tissues, prevents degeneration of epithelium lining the alimentary tract mucosa, lacrimal glands and salivary glands as well as urinary tracts.

Keywords: carotenoids, skin ageing process, UV radiation

---

* Corresponding Author Email: Joanna Igielska-Kalwat, Adam Mickiewicz University, Umultowska Street 89b, 61-614 Poznan, e-mail: joanna.igielska@amu.edu.pl, phone number: +48501667270.

Introduction

According to recent canons of beauty, the skin touched by the sun signifies healthy lifestyle and wellbeing. Unfortunately, apart from the desired nice skin tone, exposure to UV radiation and even more excessive and prolonged exposure to it, brings a whole range of undesired consequences.

UV radiation induces degenerative changes in cells of the skin, fibrous tissue and blood vessels leading to premature skin aging (Zegarska, Woźniak, 2006). The skin ageing is an unavoidable biological and psychological process studied for a long time, defined as a complex of changes taking place with time. The changes include reduction in biological activity of the cells, slowing down of regeneration processes, weakening of natural resistance and slowing down the responses to environmental stress and weakening of the adaptability of the organism controlled by genetic factors. These changes make the human organism more susceptible to damage or diseases (Batko, 2005), (Kopczewska, Kopczewski, 2005).

The skin makes an excellent model to study the process of ageing. It is directly exposed to destructive effect of the elements and hence more prone to ageing than other organs of the body. Understanding of the mechanisms of ageing is vital for developing methods delaying this process. Ageing is a multifactorial process controlled by both genetic and environmental factors. From the genetic side the process of ageing is controlled by the complex of genes responsible for cell division, antioxidative DNA repair and immunological protection (Olek-Hrab, Hawrylak et al., 2008), (Rouger, 1990), (Ramos-e-Silva, Coelho da Silca Carneiro, 2006) (Figure 1).

There are several types of the skin ageing process.

1. intrinsic;
2. chronological, hormonal (related to menopause), mimic ageing (mioageing);
3. extrinsic or photoageing controlled by external factors
4. UV-photoageing related to excessive exposure to UV radiation (Zegarska, Woźniak, 2006).

Skin ageing process

Causes of intrinsic ageing
- Genetic conditions
- Dysfunction of the neuroendocrinic system
- Weakening of immunological system
- Destructive effect of free radicals
- Accumulation of toxins in the organism

Causes of extrinsic ageing
- Damaging effect of sunlight
- Pollution of natural environment
- Climate
- Improper lifestyle
- Improper eating
- Improper skin care
- stress
- infections

Figure 1. The main causes of skin ageing (Mossakowska, Więcek, Błedowski, 2006).

Causes of the Skin Ageing

Photoageing can be treated as the process of gradual cicatrisation, intensified by other environmental factors such as smoking, air pollution, lack of sleep, improper diet, hormonal agents and diseases.

Both, beneficial and damaging effects of sunlight on the skin are related to the influence of electromagnetic radiation. Thc full spectrum of solar radiation includes infrared radiation of the wavelength longer than 800nm, visible light of the wavelengths from the range 400-800nm and ultraviolet radiation (UV) which is divided into three subranges denoted as UVC, UVB and UVA related to different biological effects. UVC radiation of the wavelengths 100-290 nm in standard conditions does not reach the Earth surface as it is almost entirely absorbed by the ozone layer. The radiation from this range is responsible for damaging the eye cornea, it has bactericidal properties and causes erythema. UVB radiation of the wavelengths 290-320 nm causes sunburn, while UVA of the wavelength from the range 320-400 nm is responsible for immediate skin colouration and delayed reactions. There are two subranges UVA1 (340-400 nm) and UVA2 (320-340 nm) they are responsible for erythema and colouration. UVA radiation makes 90-95% of sun radiation reaching the Earth (Callaghan, Wilhelm, 2008), (Augustyniak, Skrzydlewska 2004), (Yaar, Gilchrest 2001), (Gosain, Di Pietro 2004). About 50% of UVA penetrates through the reticular and papillary layers of dermis, while UVB is in 90% absorbed by the corneal layer of epidermis (Rouger, 1990). Biological effects of UV irradiation on the skin depend on the intensity and wavelength. The early reactions are erythema and sunburn, while the delayed effects are related to the damage on molecular level and include disturbed pigmentation, development of zmian przedrakowych and tumours (Żakowska-Wachelko, Pędich 1995), (Gilhar et al., 2004), (Dean, Morgan, 1998).

The clinical image of premature skin ageing comprises the appearance of wrinkles and coarse wrinkles, overdrying and abnormal keratinocyte maturation, discolouration (mottled hyperpigmentation), teleangiectasia with hypertrophic changes such as solar keratosis and seborrhoetic keratosis and reduction of skin elasticity (Giacomoni, Rein, 2004). UVA enhances the effect of UVB in the epidermis but also damages the connective tissue (Rouger, 1990), (Ramos-e-Silva, Coelho da Silca Carneiro, 2006). The effects of UVA in dermis include disturbances to microcirculation and angiogenesis and fragmentation of elastic fibres (Yu et al., 1996).

Carotenoids

Carotenoids, which belong to the best known natural antioxidants, have been for many years the subject of studies aimed at their possible application in cosmetic industry (Baran, Maibach, 1998), (Gryszczyńska, 2002). So far over 700 carotenoids have been identified, 60 of them are found in everyday diet and 20 can be detected in the blood (Anderson 2009).

Carotenoids contain 11 coupled double bonds, so they can be classified as polyisoprenoids and they are weakly polar (Fratianni et al., 2010). They can be found in acyclic, monocyclic or bicyclic form. In contrast to plants, animals are not able to synthesise carotenoids via biochemical processes, so these substances have to be provided with food (Geens et al., 2009).

Carotenoids are the yellow, orange, red or sometimes violet plant dyes. In plants they occur together with chlorophyll in chloroplasts or separately in chromoplasts. They are responsible for colouring of different parts of plants, usually flowers and fruit, rarely roots. As in the cells chlorophyll is decomposed earlier than carotene, carotenoids remain longer in ageing leaves and are responsible for characteristic autumn colours (Juola, 2008). Carotenes are orange dyes from the group of carotenoids, their main representatives are α-, β-, γ- carotene, α- and γ- carotene in the presence of carotenase are transformed into one molecule of vitamin A, while β-carotene is transformed in two molecules of vitamin A, and lycopene found in tomatoes (Baran, 1998), (Gryszczyńska et al., 2002).

Xanthophylls are yellow or yellow-orange dyes from the group of carotenoids. Chemically, xanthophylls are tetraterpenes of much greater structural diversity than carotenes. They are widespread in lower and higher plants in which they occur separately or together with chlorophyll and are responsible for the colouring of flowers, fruit and seeds. Xanthophylls include capsorubin and capsanthin, the main dyes of mature fruit of paprika, and fucoxsanthin occurring in diatoms and brown algae in so large amounts that it masks chlorophyll and dyes the chromatophores brown. Similarly as carotenes, xanthophylls protect against excessive exposure to sunlight (Christaki, 2013).

Carotenoids showing antioxidising properties include also zeaxanthine present in maize, rosa canina and common sea-buckthorn, crocetin present in the flowers of verbascum and in saffron, cryptoxanthine occurring in the citrus fruit, lutein (carotenoid of algae, present also in spinach, savoy cabbage, maize and broccoli) eliminating peroxide radicals, neoxanthine present in spinach (inhibits production of peroxides and prevents the attachment of the chemical carcinogen DMBA to DNA, inhibits carcinogensis at the stage of initiation and post-initiation (Iturriga et al., 2002).

Not all carotenoids are precursors of vitamin A, the main such precursors in the diet are β- and α- carotene. Proper intake of these precursors prevents the insufficiency of vitamin A and health problems related to it. To become active, carotenes must be converted to retinol. Almost half of absorbed carotenes undergo this conversion but only 15% of them are used by human organism (Rock, 2011).

Provitamin A assists in regeneration of tissues, prevents degeneration of epithelium lining the alimentary tract mucosa, lacrimal glands and salivary glands as well as urinary tracts (Rock et al., 2007).

In the cells of living organisms carotenoids occur mostly in complexes with proteins and they act as antioxidants. Recently, the interest in oxidation processes related to ageing as well as many diseases, has much increased. The increased intensity of oxidation processes has been observed in people in advanced age. The activity of carotenoids as antioxidants is mainly related to the possibility of absorption of some energy of oxygen in the singlet state as a result of which it transits to a state of lower energy, which means that carotenoids quench singlet oxygen, (Rodríguez-Bernaldo, de Quirós, Costa, 2006). It is possible thanks to the conjugated double bonds capable of absorption of light. Some carotenoids contain a cyclohexane ring with hydroxyl substituents or ketone groups, e.g., in cantaxanthine or astaxanthine. The mechanisms of antioxidising activity of carotenoids are related to their ability to photoprotection, capturing of free oxygen radicals and effective scavenging of peroxyl radicals. The high ability of astaxanthine to scavenge free radicals, higher than that of β-carotene, can be explained by inducing by the ketone group present in astaxanthine ring, great changes in electron density near the ends of the polyene chain of its molecule. It helps to stabilise the molecule after transition to the radical state. Carotenoids are also capable of termination of chain reactions (Sikora, 2005). It is probably possible by attachment of peroxyl lipid radical to the conjugated chain of carotenoid molecule, which leads to formation of carotenoids free radicals. Under low pressure of oxygen, the radical is able to attach one more peroxyl lipid radical and get transformed into the inactive product. Under high pressure of oxygen, instead of termination of the process, the carotenoid radical reacts with oxygen making carotenoid peroxyl radicals, so it behaves as an oxidant (Rivera S. M., Canela-Garayoa, 2012).

The properties of carotenoids as the natural antioxidants can be used in many ways in cosmetics.

Antiaging and Rejuvenating Activity of Carotenoids can be Described as Follows

- Carotenoids stimulate fibroblasts (the connective tissue cells producing protein fibres making the tissues, e.g., in the skin) to synthesise collagen and elastin, which leads to smoothing wrinkles, including deep wrinkles, crow feet around the eyes and mimic wrinkles, to increased skin density, elasticity and firmness (Anunciato, Filho, 2012),
- Carotenoids repair and regenerate collagen and elastin fibres damaged by UV radiation, leading to skin thickening and renovation (Ganceviciere et al., 2012),

- They strongly inhibit activity of elastase, the enzymes involved in degradation of collagen and elastin, so protect the skin against the loss of firmness and premature wrinkles (Fisher, 2005).
- They stimulate and normalise the process of regeneration of keratinised and UV-damaged epidermis, giving smooth and soft skin; they enhance protective effect of epidermis and reduce the through-epidermis water loss (TEWL), leading to correct hydration of epidermis which gets smooth, firm and elastic (Wilhelm et al., 1991).
- Carotenoids protect the skin against the damaging effect of free radicals whose activity contributes to premature skin ageing through degradation of collagen, elastin and fibrillin) (Anunciato, Filho, 2012),
- They stimulate natural mechanisms protecting the skin against UV radiation enhance skin resistance and support healing processes,
- They normalise the work of sebaceous glands, improve lipid management in dry and oily skin (Fisher, 2005).

Depigmentation Activity

- Carotenoids reduce the size of melanocytes and reduce the amount of melanin, which is the skin pigment that when produced in excess leads to undesired discolorations. Carotenoids considerably reduce the discolorations caused by UV radiation or hormones (minimum time of treatment – 6 months), (Cevenini et al., 2008).
- Carotenoids also reduce the post-inflammatory discolouration, e.g., post-acne discolorations (Cevenini et al., 2008).

Anti-Acne Properties

- Carotenoids are scavengers of free radicals that attack lipid components of sebum leading to generation of skin-irritating and inflammation (acne) inducing products (Naguib Yousry, 2000),
- Carotenoids normalise the work of sebaceous glands, the skin becomes less oily and shows reduced tendency to formation of comedos and eczemas (Han, 2012),

- Carotenoids clean the outlets of hair follicle, leading to narrowing of skin pores (Rice- Evans et.al., 1997),
- Carotenoids regulate and accelerate epidermis exfoliation, preventing the appearance of new acne changes (Rice- Evans et.al., 1997), (Han, 2012), (Naguib Yousry, 2000), (Igielska-Kalwat et al., 2012).

The carotenoids most often used in cosmetic industry are characterised below.

β-Carotene

Beta-carotene is applied for the treatment of photosensitivity in the patients with protoporphyria. It alleviates symptoms of acute or chronic photodamage (Igielska-Kalwat et al., 2012). β-carotene is used as an ingredient of cosmetics regulating sebum secretion. It shows anti-acne activity, softens epidermis, has anti-ageing properties and reduces the effects of photoageing (excessive keratinisation) (Staniszek, Goździcka-Józefiak, 2011). Administration of β- carotene in a dose of 30 mg/day for 10 weeks results in enhanced yellow colouration of the skin all over the body and reduction of erythema. Application of preparations with β-carotene before skin exposure to sunlight reduces the risk of sunburn because of decreased absorption of sunlight through the skin (Mączka, Wińska, 2011), (Bojarowicz, Płowiec, 2010).

Lutein and Zeaxanthine

Lutein and zeaxanthine protect the skin against premature ageing stimulated by UV exposure. They protect against the effects of UV radiation by neutralisation of triplet states of photosensitizers and singlet states of oxygen. They are antioxidants towards the reactive forms of oxygen and nitrogen. Moreover, they absorb blue light that is considered as more damaging than UV radiation and eliminate the effect of grey skin. They are recommended for the ageing skin covered with multiple wrinkles (Morganti et al., 2012).

Lycopene

Lycopene is used in creams protecting the skin against UV radiation, revitalising and regenerating. It has many beneficial effects on the skin. It helps maintain correct skin density and firmness, it is involved in the synthesis of procollagen, which is the precursor of collagen that is responsible for skin elasticity and protects hyaluronic acid against decomposition. Extracts from tomatoes are used in creams of revitalising effects, regenerative and firmness inducing activity, recommended for dry, grey and tired skin. Extracts from tomatoes can also be used for cleansing of oily skin (Darvin et al., 2011), (Igielska-Kalwat et al., 2014).

Astaxanthine

Astaxanthine is an effective absorbent of UV radiation, so it protects against erythema, photoageing, changes in DNA induced by free radicals. It is a very popular ingredient of creams with UV filters. Astaxanthine slows down the oxidising processes that destroy lipids and phospholipid cell membranes, therefore it is recommended not just for facial skin but for the whole body. It protects collagen against decomposition and hence prevents the appearance of wrinkles. It also reduces the content of melanin in the skin, so reduces the risk of the appearance of freckles, melasma and other discolourations and endows the skin with nice and homogeneous colouring (Arakane, 2010), (Capelli, 2007), (Igielska-Kalwat, 2013).

Conclusion

High concentrations of carotenoids in the skin are related to the stress-free lifestyle and use of supplementation products with carotenoids. Low concentration of carotenoids is related to unhealthy lifestyle, improper diet, smoking and diseases. Kinetics of carotenoids degradation is very fast (a few hours), while the regeneration of the skin takes at least a few days. In view of the above, the protection of skin against oxidative stress is an important problem that may be alleviated thanks to the application of cosmetic products rich in carotenoids (Alvarez et al., 2014). Carotenoids have been of considerable interest to modern cosmetic industry and at resent many cosmetic laboratories work on the best ways of using the multifarious beneficial properties of these plant dyes.

REFERENCES

[1] Zegarska B., Woźniak M (2006) Przyczyny wewnątrzpochodnego starzenia się skóry. *Gerontologia Polska* 14:153-159.

[2] Batko J (2005) Mechanizm procesu starzenia się. Nasza droga do kosmetologii. *WSZPZiUP* 2: 209-15.

[3] Kopczewska M, Kopczewski B (2005) Apoptoza- genetycznie zaprogramowana śmierć komórki. *Nowiny Lekarskie* 73: 389-92.

[4] Olek-Hrab K, Hawrylak A, Czarnecka - Operacz M (2008) Wybrane zagadnienia z zakresu starzenia się skóry. *Postep Derm i Alergol* 5: 226-234.

[5] Rouger A (1990) Czy promieniowanie UV jest niebezpieczne? *Postęp Derm i Alergol 7*: 351-357.

[6] Mossakowsa M, Więcek A, Błędowski P (2006) Aspekty medyczne, psychologicne, socjologiczne I ekonomicznes tarzenia się ludzi w Polsce. *Termedia Wydawnictwo Medyczne*. Poznań.

[7] Ramos-e-Silva M, Coelho da Silca Carneiro S (2006) Elderly skin and its rejuvenation: products and procedures for the aging skin. *IACD* 6: 40-50.

[8] Callaghan TM, Wilhelm KP (2008) A review of ageing and an examination of clinical methods in the assessment of ageing skin. Part I: Cellular and molecular perspectives of skin ageing. *Int J Cosmetic Sci* 30: 313-322.

[9] Augustyniak A, Skrzydlewska E (2004)Zdolności antyoksydacyjne w starzejącym się organizmie. *Postępy Hig Med Dosw* 58: 194-201.

[10] Yaar M, Gilchrest BA (2001) Skin aging: postulated mechanisms and consequent changes in structure and function. *Clin Geriatr Med* 17: 617-630.

[11] Gosain A, DiPietro L (2004) Aging and wound healing. *World J Surg*28: 321-326.

[12] Żakowska-Wachelko B, Pędich W (1995) Pacjenci w starszym wieku. *PZWL*, Warszawa.

[13] Gilhar A, Ullmann Y, Karry R et al., (2004) Ageing of human epidermis:the role of apoptosis. Fas and telomerase. *Br J Dermatol* 150: 56-63.
[14] Dean W, Morgan RF (1998) In defense of the concept of biological aging measurement: current status. *Arch Gerontol. Geriatr* 7: 191-210.
[15] Giacomoni PU, Rein G (2004) A mechanistic model for the aging ofhuman skin. *Micron* 35: 179-184.
[16] Yu CE, Oshima J, Fu YH. et al., (1996) Positional cloning of the Werner's syndrome gene. *Science* 272: 258-262.
[17] Andersson SC (2009) Carotenoids, tocochromanols and chlorophylls in sea buckthorn berries and rose hips. *Doctoral Thesis Swedish University of Agricultural Sciences*, Alnarp.
[18] Fratianni A, Cinquanta L, Panfili G (2010) Degradation of carotenoids In Orange juice Turing microwave heating. *Food Sci Technol* 43: 71-867.
[19] Geens A, Dauwe T, Eans M (2009) Does antropogenicmetal pollution affect carotenoids colouration, antioxidative capacity and physiological condition of great tits. *Comp Biochem Physiol* 63: 150-155.
[20] Juola F. A. McGraw K, Dearborn DC (2008) Carotenoids and throat pouch coloration in the great frigate bird. *Comp Biochem Physiol* 149: 370-7.
[21] Baran R, Maibach H (1998) *Textbook of cosmetic dermatology*, London.
[22] Gryszczyńska A, Gryszczyńska B, Opala B (2002) Karotenoidy. Naturalne źródła, biosynteza, wpływ na organizm ludzki. *Postep Fitote* 2: 127-143.
[23] Christaki E, Bonos E, Giannenas I, Florou-Paneri P (2013) Functional properties of carotenoids originating from algae. *J Sci Food Agric* 93: 5-11.
[24] Iturriga A., Velayos A, Eslava AP (2000)Structure and Function of the Genes Involved in the Biosynthesis of carotenoids in the mucorales. *Biotechnol Bioprocess Eng*. 5: 263-274.
[25] Rock ChL (2011) Carotenoids, biology and treatment. *Pharmacol Ther* 3: 185-197.
[26] Rock H, Braun Ch L, Ernst H (2007) The Chemistry of Novel Xanthophyll Carotenoids. *The American Journal of Cardiology* 10: 51-57.
[27] Rodríguez-Bernaldo de Quirós A, Costa HS (2006) Analysis of carotenoids in vegetable and plasma samples: a review. *J Food Compos Anal* 19: 97-111.

[28] Sikora M (2005) Karotenoidy, wielofunkcyjne składniki preparatów kosmetycznych. *Magazyn Partnerów Polskiej Grupy Farmaceutycznej "Bez Recepty"* 5: 17-19.

[29] Rivera S., Canela-Garayoa R (2012) Analytical tools for the analysis of carotenoids in diverse materials. *Journal of Chromatography A 1224*: 1-10.

[30] Anunciato TP, Filho PA de Rocha (2012) Carotenoids and polyphenols in nutricosmetics, nutraceuticals, and cosmeceuticals *Journal of Cosmetic Dermatology* 11: 51-54.

[31] Ganceviviere R, Liakou A, Theodoridis A, Makrantonaki E (2012) Skin anti-aging strategies, *Dermato Endocrinol* 3: 308-319.

[32] Fisher, GJ (2005) The pathophysiology of photoaging of the skin. *Cutis* 5: 58–69.

[33] Wilhelm KP, Cua AB, Howard I Maibach MD (1991) Skin Aging Effect on Transepidermal Water Loss, Stratum Corneum Hydration, Skin Surface pH, and Casual Sebum Content, *Arch Dermatol* 12:1806-1809.

[34] Invidia L, Lescai F, Salvioli S, Tieri P, Castellani G, et al., (2008) Human models of aging and longevity. *Expert Opin Biol The* 8: 1393–405

[35] Naguib Yousry MA (2000) Antioxidant activities of astaxanthin and related carotenoids. *J Agric Food Chem* 48: 1150-1154.

[36] Han RM, Zhang JP., Skibsted LH (2012) Reaction Dynamics of Flavonoids and Carotenoids as Antioxidants. *Molecule*s 17: 2140-2160.

[37] Rice - Evans C, Miller N, Paganga G (1997) Antioxidant properties of phenolic compounds. *Trends Plant Sci 2, 152-159.*

[38] Igielska-Kalwat J, Wawrzyńczak A, Nowak I (2012) Karotenoidy i ich zastosowanie w przemyśle kosmetycznym. *Chemik* 2, 140-144.

[39] Staniszek K, Goździcka-Józefiak A (2008) Wpływ β-karotenu, retinoidów i receptorów retinoidowych na proliferację i transformację nowotworową komórek. *Biotechnologia* 3: 28-45.

[40] Mączka W, Wińska K (2011) β-karoten – przyjaciel czy wróg? *Postępy Kosmetologii* 4: 259-262.

[41] Bojarowicz H, Płowiec A (2010) Wpływ witaminy A na kondycję skóry. *Prob Hig Epidemiol* 91: 352-356.

[42] Morganti P, Martins D, Morganti G (2012)Aktywność Luteiny w skórze. *SOFW- Journal* 1:13-18.

[43] Darvin E., Sterry W, Lademann J, Vergou T (2011) The Role of Carotenoids in Human Skin. *Molecules* 16:10491-10506.

[44] Igielska-Kalwat J, Gościańska J, Nowak I (2014) Zastosowanie likopenu w dermo kosmetykach. *Przemysł Chemiczny* 7: 1110-1130.

[45] Arakane K (2010) Superior Skin Protection via Astaxanthin. *Research & Development Division. KOSE Corporation.*

[46] Capelli B, przy współpracy dr Cysewskiego GR (2007) Astaksantyna. Naturalna astaksantyna- królowa karotenoidów. *Cyanotech Corporation.*

[47] Igielska-Kalwat J, Gościańska J, Nowak I (2013) Astaksantyna cenny składnik preparatów kosmetycznych. *Kosmet Estet* 2: 83-85.

[48] Alvarez R, Vaz B, Gronemeyer H, de Lera AG (2014) Functions, therapeutic applications, and synthesis of retinoids and carotenoids. *Chem Rev*; dx.doi.org/10.1021/cr400126u.

Bibliography

An evidence-based approach to phytochemicals and other dietary factors

LCCN	2012041613
Type of material	Book
Personal name	Higdon, Jane.
Main title	An evidence-based approach to phytochemicals and other dietary factors / Jane Higdon, PhD, Linus Pauling Institute, Oregon State University, Corvallis, Oregon, USA, Victoria J. Drake, PhD, Manager, Micronutrient Information Center, Linus Pauling Institute, Oregon State University, Corvallis, Oregon, USA.
Edition	2nd ed.
Published/Created	Stuttgart: Thieme, c2013.
Description	xxiv, 304 pages: illustrations; 25 cm
ISBN	9783131418425 (hardcover: alk. paper) 9783131697127 (eISBN)
LC classification	QP144.V44 H54 2013
Related names	Drake, Victoria (Victoria J.) Higdon, Jane. Evidence-based approach to dietary phytochemicals.
Summary	"Now in a completely updated second edition, An Evidence-based Approach to Dietary Phytochemicals and Other Dietary Factors is a trusted resource for all health professionals who need to interpret the explosion of information on the role of a plant-based diet in health and disease. It consolidates a wealth of

scientifically accurate, peer-reviewed data on plant foods, dietary phytochemicals, and dietary supplements, and includes information on essential intake recommendations, dietary sources, nutrient and drug interactions, phytochemicals in disease prevention, possible adverse effects, and much more. Special features: All chapters revised and updated, with new sections on choline, coenzyme Q10, L-Carnitine, lipoic acid, and other dietary factors Logically structured for quick access to information--begins with the evidence-based benefits of fruits and vegetables, legumes, nuts, whole grains, coffee, and tea; and goes on to the scientific and clinical data on individual dietary phytochemicals and classes of phytochemicals, including carotenoids, flavonoids, fiber, and more Summaries at the end of each chapter for rapid review Peer-reviewed by experts in the field, ensuring that all material is accurate and up-to-date The well-constructed appendix includes not only a quick reference to diseases and foods and where to find them in the book; but also useful tables on phytochemical-drug interactions, phytochemical-nutrient interactions, and phytochemical-rich foods; a summary of the glycemic index of dietary carbohydrates; and a comprehensive glossary of terms"-- Provided by publisher.

Subjects	Plant Extracts--therapeutic use.
	Dietary Supplements.
	Phytotherapy--methods.
	Plants, Edible--chemistry.
Notes	Rev. ed. of: An evidence-based approach to dietary phytochemicals / Jane Higdon. c2007.
	Includes bibliographical references and index.

Bioactive foods in promoting health. Fruits and vegetables

LCCN	2013444243
Type of material	Book
Main title	Bioactive foods in promoting health. Fruits and vegetables / edited by Ronald Ross Watson, Victor R.

	Preedy.
Edition	1st ed.
Published/Created	London; Burlington, MA: Academic Press, 2010.
Description	xvi, 737 p.: ill.; 25 cm.
ISBN	9780123746283 (hbk.) 0123746280 (hbk.)
LC classification	QP144.F85 B533 2010
Variant title	Fruits and vegetables
Related names	Watson, Ronald R. (Ronald Ross) Preedy, Victor R.
Summary	"While everyone knows fruits and vegetables are beneficial to good health, it's increasingly seen as important to know which ones can be effective in treating specific illnesses. Bioactive Foods in Promoting Health: Fruits and Vegetables brings together experts working on the different aspects of supplementation, foods, and plant extracts, in health promotion and disease prevention. Their expertise and experience provide the most current knowledge to promote future research. Dietary habits need to be altered, for most people and the conclusions and recommendations from the various chapters in this book will provide a basis for that change. The overall goal of this book is to provide the most current, concise, scientific appraisal of the efficacy of key foods and constituents medicines in dietary plants in preventing disease and improving the quality of life. While vegetables have traditionally been seen to be good sources of vitamins, the roles of other constituents have only recently become more widely recognized. This book reviews and often presents new hypotheses and conclusions on the effects of different bioactive components of the diet, derived particularly from vegetables, to prevent disease and improve the health of various populations."--Publisher's description.
Contents	Sect. A. Fruit and Vegetables in Health Promotion -- 1. Botanical Diversity in Vegetable and Fruit Intake: Potential Health Benefits / Matthew D. Thompson and

Henry J. Thompson -- 2. Vegetable and Fruit Intake and the Development of Cancer: A Brief Review and Analysis / Henry J. Thompson -- 3. Fruit and Vegetable Antioxidants in Health / Manuela Blasa, Lorenzo Gennari, Donato Angelino and Paolino Ninfali -- 4. Medicinal Activities of Essential Oils: Role in Disease Prevention / Alfreda Wei and Takayuki Shibamoto -- 5. Emerging Knowledge of the Bioactivity of Foods in the Diets of Indigenous North Americans / Alexander G. Schauss -- 6. Barriers and Facilitating Factors Affecting Fruit and Vegetable Consumption / Ming-Chin Yeh, Janel Obenchain and Anahi Viladrich -- 7. Healthy Eating: What Is the Role of the Economic Situation? / Tea Lallukka, Mikko Laaksonen and Ossi Rahkonen -- 8. Trends in US Adult Fruit and Vegetable Consumption / Sarah Stark Casagrande and Tiffany L. Gary-Webb -- 9. Fruit and Vegetables in the Optimized Mixed Diet / Ute Alexy and Mathilde Kersting -- 10. Antibacterial Properties of Dietary Fruit / Rachel O'Mahony -- 11. Fruit and Vegetable Intake of Mothers in Europe: Risks/Benefits / Alexandra Wolf and Ibrahim Elmadfa -- 12. Fruit, Vegetables, and Bone Health / Yu Ming Chen and Suzanne C. Ho -- 13. Socioeconomic Inequalities in Fruit and Vegetable Intakes / Kylie Ball and David Crawford -- 14. Working with Industry for the Promotion of Fruit and Vegetable Consumption / Christina M. Pollard and Chris Rowley -- Sect. B. Effects of Individual Vegetables on Health -- 15. Garlic and Aging: Current Knowledge and Future Considerations / Carmia Borek -- 16. Garlic and Heart Health / Khalid Rahman -- 17. Fig, Carob, Pistachio, and Health / Soliman Khatib and Jacob Vaya -- 18. Poi History, Uses, and Role in Health / Salam A. Ibrahim and Danfeng Song -- 19. Increasing Children's Liking and Intake of Vegetables through Experiential Learning / Remco C. Havermans -- 20. Bioactivity of Polyacetylenes in Food Plants / Lars P. Christensen -- 21. Nitrates and Nitrites in Vegetables: Occurrence and

Health Risks / Terje Tamme, Mari Reinik and Mati Roasto -- 22. Essentiality of Nutritional Supplementation in HIV Infection and AIDS: Review of Clinical Studies and Results from a Community Health Micronutrient Program / Raxit J. Jariwalla, Alexandra Niedzwiecki and Matthias Rath -- 23. Tomatoes, Tomato Products, and Lycopene in Prevention and Therapy of Prostate Diseases: Is There Evidence from Intervention Studies for Preventive and for Therapeutic Effects? / Sabine Ellinger -- 24. Fruit, Vegetables, and Legumes Consumption: Role in Preventing and Treating Obesity / Ana B. Crujeiras, Estibalíz Goyenechea and J. Alfredo Martínez -- 25. Spinach and Carrots: Vitamin A and Health / Guangwen Tang -- 26. Spinach and Health: Anticancer Effect / Naoki Maeda, Hiromi Yoshida and Yoshiyuki Mizushina -- 27. Potential Health Benefits of Rhubarb / Elisabetta M. Clementi and Francesco Misiti -- 28. Health Benefits of Fenugreek (Trigonella foenum-graecum leguminosse) / Tapan K. Basu and Anchalee Srichamroen -- 29. Weight Loss Due to Fruit and Vegetable Use / Elena Rodríguez-Rodríguez, Ana M. López-Sobaler and Rosa M. Ortega -- 30. Legumes and Cardiovascular Disease / Peter M. Clifton -- Sect. C. Actions of Individual Fruits in Disease and Cancer Prevention and Treatment -- 31. Biological Effects of Pomegranate (Punica granatum L.), especially its Antibacterial Actions, Against Microorganisms Present in the Dental Plaque and Other Infectious Processes / Glauce S.B. Viana, Silvana Magalhães Siqueira Menezes, Luciana N. Cordeiro and F.J.A. Matos -- 32. Açaí (Euterpe oleracea Mart.): A Macro and Nutrient Rich Palm Fruit from the Amazon Rain Forest with Demonstrated Bioactivities In Vitro and In Vivo / Alexander G. Schauss -- 33. Beneficial uses of Breadfruit (Artocarpus altilis): Nutritional, Medicinal and Other Uses / Neela Badrie and Jacklyn Broomes -- 34. Bioactive Compounds in Mango (Mangifera indica L.) / Sônia Machado Rocha Ribeiro and Andreas

	Schieber -- 35. Health Benefits of Bitter Melon (Momordica charantia) / Edralin A. Lucas, Gerard G. Dumancas, Brenda J. Smith, Stephen L. Clarke and Bahram H. Arjmandi -- 36. Pomegranate in Human Health: An Overview / Ana Faria and Conceição Calhau -- 37. Kiwifruit and Health / Denise C. Hunter, Margot A. Skinner, A. Ross Ferguson and Lesley M. Stevenson -- 38. Bioactive Chemicals and Health Benefits of Grapevine Products / Marcello Iriti and Franco Faoro -- 39. Soursop (Annona muricata L.): Composition, Nutritional Value, Medicinal Uses, and Toxicology / Neela Badrie and Alexander G. Schauss -- 40. Carotenoids in Vegetables: Biosynthesis, Occurrence, Impacts on Human Health, and Potential for Manipulation / Dean A. Kopsell and David E. Kopsell -- 41. Apigenin and Cancer Chemoprevention / Sanjeev Shukla and Sanjay Gupta -- 42. Goitrogen in Food: Cyanogenic and Flavonoids Containing Plant Foods in the Development of Goiter / Amar K. Chandra -- 43. Nutritional and Health Benefits of Root Crops / Trinidad P. Trinidad, Aida C. Mallillin, Anacleta C. Loyola, Rosario R. Encabo and Rosario S. Sagum.
Subjects	Functional foods. Vegetables in human nutrition. Fruit in human nutrition. Fruit. Vegetables. Health Promotion. Neoplasms--prevention & control. Nutrition Therapy. Nutritional Physiological Phenomena. Fruit in human nutrition. Functional foods. Vegetables in human nutrition.
Notes	Includes bibliographical references and index.

Biosynthesis and molecular genetics of fungal secondary metabolites

LCCN	2014946216
Type of material	Book
Main title	Biosynthesis and molecular genetics of fungal secondary metabolites / Juan-Francisco Martin, Carlos García-Estrada, Susanne Zeilinger, editors.
Published/Produced	New York: Springer, [2014]
Description	volumes: illustrations (some color); 24 cm.
Links	Table of contents http://catdir.loc.gov/catdir/enhancements/fy1412/2014946216-t.html Contributor biographical information http://catdir.loc.gov/catdir/enhancements/fy1412/2014946216-b.html Publisher description http://catdir.loc.gov/catdir/enhancements/fy1412/2014946216-d.html
ISBN	9781493911905 (v. 1: alk. paper) 1493911902 (v. 1: alk. paper) 9781493911912 (v. 1: eBook) 1493911910 (v. 1: eBook) 9781493925308 (v. 2: alk. paper) 149392530X (v. 2: alk. paper) (v. 2: eBook)
LC classification	QK601 .B56 2014
Related names	Martín, Juan Francisco, editor. García-Estrada, Carlos, editor. Zeilinger, Susanne, editor.
Summary	This volume describes the more relevant secondary metabolites of different fungi with current information on their biosynthesis and molecular genetics. Bolstered with color illustrations and photographs, the book describes the possible application of molecular genetics to directed strain improvement in great detail. The needs for future developments in this field are also discussed at length. Written by authorities in the field, Biosynthesis and Molecular Genetics of Fungal Secondary Metabolites provides a cutting-edge perspective on fungal secondary metabolism and underlying genetics and is a valuable resource for scientists, researchers, and educators in the field of fungal biology.-- Source other than Library of

	Congress.
Contents	Valuable Secondary Metabolites from Fungi -- Penicillins -- Cephalosporins -- Cyclosporines: Biosynthesis and Beyond -- Aflatoxin Biosynthesis: Regulation and Subcellular Localization -- Roquefortine C and Related Prenylated Indole Alkaloids -- Ochratoxin A and Related Mycotoxins -- Carotenoids -- Astaxanthin and Related Xanthophylls -- Gibberellins and the Red Pigments Bikaverin and Fusarubin -- Fusarins and Fusaric Acid in Fusaria -- Lovastatin, Compactin, and Related Anticholesterolemic Agents -- Meroterpenoids -- Ergot Alkaloids -- Fungal NRPS-dependent Siderophores: from Function to Prediction.
Subjects	Fungal metabolites. Biosynthesis. Metabolism, Secondary. Fungi--metabolism Fungi--genetics Biological Products Metabolomics Cell Biology. Microbiology. Plant Genetics & Genomics. Plant Biochemistry. Science--Life Sciences--Anatomy & Physiology. Biosynthesis. Fungal metabolites. Metabolism, Secondary.
Notes	Includes bibliographical references and index.
Series	Fungal Biology, 2198-7777 Fungal biology (Springer (Firm)), 2198-7777

Carotenoid cleavage products

LCCN	2013022427
Type of material	Book
Main title	Carotenoid cleavage products / Peter Winterhalter, editor, Institute of Food Chemistry, Technische Universitat Braunschweig, Braunschweig, Germany,

	Susan E. Ebeler, editor, Department of Viticulture and Enology, University of California Davis, Davis, California; sponsored by the ACS Division of Agriculture and Food Chemistry, Inc.
Published/Produced	Washington, DC: American Chemical Society, [2013]
Description	x, 238 pages; 24 cm.
ISBN	9780841227781 (hbk.: alkaline paper)
LC classification	QK898.C34 C36 2013
Related names	Winterhalter, Peter, 1957- Ebeler, Susan E., 1961- American Chemical Society. Division of Agricultural and Food Chemistry.
Contents	[I] Bio-Oxidative Cleavage -- Carotenoid cleavage products: an introduction -- Carotenoid cleavage dioxygenase genes from fruit -- Involvement of CCD4 in determining petal color -- Carotenoid cleavage dioxygenase and presence of apo-carotenoids in biological matrices -- [II] Aroma-Active Carotenoid Metabolites -- Carotenoid cleavage products in saffron (Crocus sativus l.) -- Biodegradation of carotenoids: an important route to scent formation -- C13-apocarotenoids: more than flavor compounds? -- Carotenoid content and flavor of pumpkin juice -- Carotenoid cleavage products in grapes and wines -- Biosynthesis of C13-norisoprenoids in Vitis vinifera: evidence of carotenoid cleavage dioxygenase (CCD) and secondary transformation of norisoprenoid compounds -- Behavior of glycosylated monoterpenes, C13-norisoprenoids, and benzenoids in Vitis vinifera cv. Riesling during ripening and following hedging -- TDN and [beta]-Damascenone: two important carotenoid metabolites in wine -- Monitoring carotenoids and derivative compounds in grapes and port wines: impact on quality -- [III] Biotechnology and Processing Effects -- Biotechnological production of norisoprenoid aroma compounds -- Design of aqueous micellar reaction systems for aroma production with carotenoid cleavage dioxygenase -- In situ product recovery of [beta]-ionone by organophilic

	pervaporation -- Oxidative cleavage products of lycopene: production and reactivity in a biomimetic experimental model of oxidative stress -- Intramolecular cyclisation as structural transformation of carotenoids during processing of paprika (Capsicum annuum l.) and paprika oleoresins -- Egg yolk carotenoids: composition, analysis, and effects of processing on their stability.
Subjects	Carotenoids--Analysis--Congresses. Carotenoids--Metabolism--Congresses. Metabolites--Congresses. Oxygenases--Congresses. Enzymes--Congresses. Food--Analysis--Congresses.
Notes	Includes bibliographical references and indexes.
Series	ACS symposium series; 1134

Carotenoids: food sources, production and health benefits

LCCN	2013944999
Type of material	Book
Main title	Carotenoids: food sources, production and health benefits / Masayoshi Yamaguchi, editor.
Published/Created	New York: Nova Publishers, c2013.
Description	xiii, 355 p.: ill. (some col.); 27 cm.
ISBN	9781628086225 162808622X
LC classification	QP671.C35 C365 2013
Related names	Yamaguchi, Masayoshi, 1947-
Subjects	Carotenoids. Carotenoids--Physiological effect.
Notes	Includes bibliographical references and index.
Series	Nutrition and diet research progress Biochemistry research trends Nutrition and diet research progress series.

Carotenoids: nutrition, analysis and technology

LCCN	2015020395
Type of material	Book
Main title	Carotenoids: nutrition, analysis and technology /

	[edited by] Agnieszka Kaczor, Malgorzata Baranska.
Published/Produced	Chichester, UK; Hoboken, New Jersey: John Wiley & Sons, 2016.
ISBN	9781118622261 (cloth)
LC classification	QP671.C35 C372 2016
Related names	Kaczor, Agnieszka, editor. Baranska, Malgorzata, editor.
Contents	Carotenoids: overview of nomenclature, structures, occurrence, and functions / A. Kaczor, M. Baranska, K. Czamara -- The role of antioxidants in prevention of premature skin aging / J. Lademann, M.E. Darvin, F. Knorr, S. Jung, L. Zastrow, M.C. Meinke -- Anti-tumor activity of dietary carotenoids: prospects for applications in therapy / H. Abramczyk, J. Surmacki -- Photo- and radiation protection of dietary carotenoids / F. Boehm, R. Edge, T. G. Truscott, C. Witt -- Macular carotenoids: human health aspects / A. Gorusupudi, P. Bernstein -- Vibrational spectroscopy as a tool to investigate carotenoids / J. Cz. Dobrowolski -- Structural studies of carotenoids in plants, animals and food products / T. Maoka -- In situ studies of carotenoids in plants and animals / M. Baranska, J. Cz. Dobrowolski, G. Zajac -- Carotenoids in pigment-protein complexes: relation between carotenoids structure and function / W. I. Gruszecki -- Carotenoid biosynthesis and regulation in plants / R. Baranski, C. I. Cazzonelli -- Carotenoids bioavailability from food matrix: towards efficient extraction procedures / H. Schulz -- Carotenoid production by bacteria, microalgae and fungi / R. M. Schweiggert, R. Carle -- Impact of stress factors on carotenoid structures and bioavailability / A. Kaczor, M. Pilarczyk -- Syntheses with carotenoids / H.-R. Sliwka, V. Partali.
Subjects	Carotenoids.
Notes	Includes bibliographical references and index.
Additional formats	Online version: Carotenoids Chichester, UK; Hoboken, New Jersey: John Wiley & Sons, 2016 9781118622247 (DLC) 2015028232

Carotenoids: physical, chemical, and biological functions and properties

LCCN	2009036998
Type of material	Book
Main title	Carotenoids: physical, chemical, and biological functions and properties / edited by John T. Landrum.
Published/Created	Boca Raton: CRC Press, c2010.
Description	xv, 544 p., [8] p. of plates: ill. (some col.); 27 cm.
ISBN	9781420052305 (hardcover: alk. paper) 1420052306 (hardcover: alk. paper)
LC classification	QP671.C35 C376 2010
Related names	Landrum, John Thomas.
Subjects	Carotenoids. Carotenoids.
Notes	Includes bibliographical references and index.
Dewey class no.	612.4/9

Carotenoids: properties, effects, and diseases

LCCN	2011038711
Type of material	Book
Main title	Carotenoids: properties, effects, and diseases / Masayoshi Yamaguchi, editor.
Published/Created	New York: Nova Science Publishers, c2010.
Description	xi, 440 p.: ill; 26 cm.
ISBN	9781612097138 (hardcover)
LC classification	QP671.C35 C373 2010
Related names	Yamaguchi, Masayoshi, 1947-
Subjects	Carotenoids--chemistry. Carotenoids--therapeutic use.
Notes	Includes bibliographical references and index.
Series	Biochemistry research trends

Carotenoids and human health

LCCN	2012951405
Type of material	Book
Main title	Carotenoids and human health / Sherry A. Tanumihardjo, editor.
Published/Produced	New York: Humana Press, [2013]
Description	xxiii, 331 pages: illustrations (some color), portraits, maps; 26 cm.

ISBN	9781627032025 (hardcover: alk. paper)
	1627032029 (hardcover: alk. paper)
LC classification	QP671.C35 C36 2013
Related names	Tanumihardjo, Sherry A., editor of compilation.
Subjects	Carotenoids--physiology.
	Nutritional Physiological Phenomena.
Notes	Includes bibliographical references and index.
Series	Nutrition and health series
	Nutrition and health (Totowa, N.J.)

Carotenoids and retinal disease

LCCN	2013030826
Type of material	Book
Main title	Carotenoids and retinal disease / edited by John T. Landrum, John M. Nolan.
Published/Produced	Boca Raton: CRC Press/Taylor & Francis Group, [2014]
Description	xxii, 242 pages, 8 colored plates: illustrations; 24 cm
ISBN	9781466502048 (hardcover: acid-free paper)
LC classification	RE661.D3 C37 2014
Related names	Landrum, John Thomas, editor of compilation.
	Nolan, John (John M.), editor of compilation.
Summary	"This book outlines the pathological conditions of the central retina where the macular pigment is known to have its greatest involvement in protection against photooxidative damage. The book focuses on the nature of the macular carotenoids, their transport and accumulation within the retina, and their influence on the etiology of retinal diseases. It also includes chapters that provide readers an understanding of the epidemiology and pathology of these diseases and the known factors which contribute to them"--Provided by publisher.
Subjects	Macular Degeneration.
	Carotenoids--analysis.
	Risk Factors.
Notes	Includes bibliographical references and index.

Carotenoids and vitamin A in translational medicine

LCCN	2012038319
Type of material	Book
Main title	Carotenoids and vitamin A in translational medicine / edited by Olaf Sommerburg, Werner Siems, and Klaus Kraemer.
Published/Created	Boca Raton, FL: CRC Press/Taylor & Francis Group, c2013.
Description	xxxii, 404 p.: ill.; 24 cm.
ISBN	9781439855263 (hardcover: alk. paper)
LC classification	QP671.C3 C376 2013
Related names	Sommerburg, Olaf. Siems, Werner. Kraemer, Klaus, 1960-
Contents	Hepatic retinoid metabolism: what is known and what is not / Jason J. Yuen, Jian Zhang Yang and William S. Blaner -- Metabolism of vitamin A in white adipose tissue and obesity / Shanmugam M. Jeyakumar ... [et al.] -- Retinoids in the treatment of psoriasis / Neil Borkar, Alan Menter -- Age-related macular degeneration and carotenoids / Nilesh Kalariya, Werner G. Siems, Frederik van Kuijk -- Lutein, zeaxanthin and vision across the lifespan / Billy R. Hammond, Jr. -- Assuring vitamin A adequacy to prevent eye and ear disorders / Tripper Sauer, Susan Emmett, Keith P. West, Jr. -- Disturbed accumulation and abnormal distribution of macular pigment in retinal disorders / Tos TJM Berendschot, Peter Charbel Issa, Thomas Theelen -- Retinol and otitis media / Akeem Olawale Lasisi -- Carotenoids and mutagenesis / P. M. Eckl ... [et al.] -- Carotenoids and vitamin A in lung cancer prevention / Anita Ratnasari Iskandar, Xiang-Dong Wang -- Is the effect of [Beta]-carotene on prostate cancer cells dependent on their androgen sensitivity? / Joanna Dulinska-Litewka ... [et al.] -- Carotenoid intake and supplementation in cancer: pro and con / W.G. Siems ... [et al.] -- Vitamin A in lung development and function / Hans-Konrad Biesalski -- Vitamin A and carotenoids in lung diseases / Olaf

	Sommerburg, Werner Siems -- Chemopreventive effects of astaxanthin on inflammatory bowel disease and inflammation-related colon carcinogenesis / Masashi Hosokawa, Yumiko Yasui -- Carotenoids in laboratory medicine / Ingolf Schimke, Michael Vogeser -- Supply of vitamin A in developing countries / Klaus Kraemer -- Vitamin A intakes are below recommendations in a significant proportion of the population in the western world / Hans-Konrad Biesalski, Barbara Trösch, Petra Weber -- Critical appraisal of vitamin A supplementation program in India / Dechenla Tshering Bhutia, Saskia De Pee -- Consequences of common genetic variations on SS-carotene cleavage for vitamin A supply / Georg Lietz, Anthony Oxley, Christine Boesch-Saadatmandi.
Subjects	Carotenoids--Therapeutic use. Vitamin A--Physiological effect. Vitamin A in the body. Vitamin A--therapeutic use. Carotenoids--therapeutic use. Translational Medical Research. Vitamin A--supply & distribution. Vitamin A Deficiency--drug therapy.
Notes	Includes bibliographical references and index.
Series	Oxidative stress and disease; 33 Oxidative stress and disease; 33.

Carotenoids in nature: biosynthesis, regulation and function

LCCN	2016947054
Type of material	Book
Personal name	Stange, Claudia.
Main title	Carotenoids in nature: biosynthesis, regulation and function / Claudia Stange.
Published/Produced	New York, NY: Springer Berlin Heidelberg, 2016.
Links	Publisher description https://www.loc.gov/catdir/enhancements/fy1619/2016947054-d.html Table of contents only https://www.loc.gov/catdir/enhancements/fy1619/2016947054-t.html
ISBN	9783319391243

Citrus: molecular phylogeny, antioxidant properties and medicinal uses

LCCN	2014016918
Type of material	Book
Main title	Citrus: molecular phylogeny, antioxidant properties and medicinal uses / editor: Khizar Hayat (Department of Chemistry, COMSATS Institute of Information Technology, Abbottabad, Pakistan).
Published/Produced	Hauppauge, New York, USA: Nova Science Publishers Inc., 2014.
ISBN	9781631179853 (hardcover)
LC classification	TX558.C5 C56 2014
Related names	Hayat, Khizar.
Contents	History, ecology and challenges of citrus production in tropical and subtropical areas / Gustavo Habermann and Marcelo Claro de Souza -- Molecular characterization of citrus cultivars: insight from recent studies / Jamila Bernardi, Adriano Marocco, Paola Caruso and Concetta Licciardello -- Citrus flavonoids: their biosynthesis, functions and genetic improvement / Sabaz Ali Khan, Rafiq Ahmad, Saeed Ahmad Asad and Muhammad Shahzad -- Advances in study of carotenoids in citrus fruit / Xiangyu Liu, Juan Li and Jiezhong Chen -- Influence of postharvest handling on antioxidant compounds of citrus fruits / Sawsen Sdiri, Alejandra Salvador, Imen Farhat, Pilar Navarro and Cristina Besada -- Prophylactic propensity of citrus phytochemicals: action and mechanisms / D. Ramful-Baboolall, V.S. Neergheen-Bhujun and T. Bahorun -- Citrus medica L. Cv Diamante: an overview on the phytochemistry and potential health benefits / Rosa Tundis, Monica R. Loizzo, Marco Bonesi and Francesco Menichini -- High doses of synephrine and octopamine activate lipolysis in human adipocytes, indicating that amines from citrus might influence adiposity / Marie-Anne Carpéné, Xavier Testar and Christian Carpéné -- Features of the insecticidal action of Citrus sinensis essential oil against Musca domestica / Yanina E. Rossi, María L. González, María C. Carpinella, Diego G. Andrione and Sara M.

	Palacios -- The potential of D(+)-limonene to improve PLA-PBH blends properties / M.P. Arrieta, J. López, A. Hernández and E. Rayón.
Subjects	Citrus fruits--Analysis. Antioxidants--Health aspects. Citrus fruits--Therapeutic use. Citrus--Phylogeny--Molecular aspects.
Notes	Includes bibliographical references and index.
Series	Botanical research and practices Botanical research and practices.

Complementary and alternative medicine sourcebook: basic consumer health information about ayurveda, acupuncture, aromatherapy, chiropractic care, diet-based therapies, guided imagery, herbal and vitamin supplements, homeopathy, hypnosis, massage, meditation, naturopathy, Pilates, reflexology, reiki, shiatsu, tai chi, traditional Chinese medicine, yoga, and other complementary and alternative medical therapies; along with statistics, tips for selecting a practitioner, treatments for specific health conditions, a glossary of related terms, and a directory of resources for additional help and information

LCCN	2010013183
Type of material	Book
Main title	Complementary and alternative medicine sourcebook: basic consumer health information about ayurveda, acupuncture, aromatherapy, chiropractic care, diet-based therapies, guided imagery, herbal and vitamin supplements, homeopathy, hypnosis, massage, meditation, naturopathy, Pilates, reflexology, reiki, shiatsu, tai chi, traditional Chinese medicine, yoga, and other complementary and alternative medical therapies; along with statistics, tips for selecting a practitioner, treatments for specific health conditions, a glossary of related terms, and a directory of resources for additional help and information / edited by Amy L. Sutton.
Edition	4th ed.
Published/Created	Detroit, MI: Omnigraphics, c2010.
Description	xvi, 669 p.: ill.; 24 cm.
ISBN	9780780810822 (hardcover: alk. paper)

	0780810821 (hardcover: alk. paper)
LC classification	R735 .C66 2010
Related names	Sutton, Amy L.
Summary	"Provides basic consumer health information about alternative and complementary medical therapies, including treatments for specific diseases and conditions. Includes index, glossary of related terms, and other resources"--Provided by publisher.
Contents	What is complementary and alternative medicine (CAM)? -- Common questions and answers about CAM -- The use of CAM in the United States -- CAM use and children -- CAM use in older adults -- Health care providers and CAM -- Insurance issues and paying for CAM treatment -- Health fraud awareness -- Use caution buying medical products online -- What are whole medical systems? -- Ayurvedic medicine -- Other indigenous medical systems -- Acupuncture -- Homeopathy -- Naturopathy -- Questions and answers about dietary supplements -- Botanical dietary supplements -- Using dietary supplements wisely -- Adolescents and supplement use -- Tips for older dietary supplement users -- Vitamin A and carotenoids -- Vitamin B_6 -- Vitamin B_{12} -- Vitamin D -- Vitamin E -- Folate (Folic acid) -- Magnesium -- Omega-3 fatty acid supplements -- Selenium -- Bone and joint health supplements -- Immune system support supplements -- Mood and brain health supplements -- Probiotics: supplements for gastrointestinal health -- Sports and energy supplements -- Supplements used for weight loss -- Biologically based therapies: an overview -- Apitherapy -- Aromatherapy and essential oils -- Diet-based therapies -- Oxygen therapy -- Mind-body medicine: an overview -- Art therapy -- Biofeedback -- Deep breathing exercises -- Feng shui -- Guided imagery and hypnosis -- Meditation -- Music therapy -- Prayer and spirituality -- Relaxation training -- Tai chi -- Yoga -- Other mind-body medicine therapies -- Manipulative and body-based therapies: an overview -- Alexander technique -- Aquatic therapy

	(Hydrotherapy) -- Chiropractic care and osteopathic manipulation -- Craniosacral therapy -- Feldenkrais method -- Massage therapy -- Pilates -- Qigong -- Reflexology -- Structural integration techniques -- Other manipulative and body-based therapies -- Energy medicine: an overview -- Magnet therapy -- Polarity therapy -- Reiki -- Shiatsu -- Therapeutic touch -- Other energy-based therapies -- Arthritis and CAM -- Asthma, allergies, and CAM -- Cancer and CAM -- Cognitive decline and CAM -- Diabetes and CAM -- Fibromyalgia and CAM -- Headache and CAM -- Heart disease and chelation therapy -- Hepatitis C and CAM -- Hormones, CAM, and aging - - Infertility and CAM -- Low back pain and CAM -- Menopausal symptoms and CAM -- Mental health care and CAM -- Sleep disorders and CAM -- Glossary of terms related to alternative and complementary medicine -- Directory of organizations that provide information about alternative and complementary medicine.
Subjects	Alternative medicine--Popular works.
Notes	Includes bibliographical references and index.
Series	Health reference series Health reference series (Unnumbered)

DeVita, Hellman, and Rosenberg's cancer: principles & practice of oncology

LCCN	2011007212
Type of material	Book
Main title	DeVita, Hellman, and Rosenberg's cancer: principles & practice of oncology / [edited by] Vincent T. DeVita Jr., Theodore S. Lawrence, Steven A. Rosenberg; associate scientific advisors, Robert A. Weinberg, Ronald A. DePinho; with 431 contributing authors.
Edition	9th ed.
Published/Created	Philadelphia: Wolters Kluwer Health/Lippincott Williams & Wilkins, c2011.
Description	xlvii, 2638 p.: ill. (some col.); 29 cm.
Links	Publisher description http://www.loc.gov/catdir/

	enhancements/fy1201/2011007212-d.html Table of contents only http://www.loc.gov/catdir/enhancements/fy1201/2011007212-t.html
ISBN	9781451105452 1451105452
LC classification	RC261 .C274 2011
Portion of title	Cancer: principles & practice of oncology
Related names	DeVita, Vincent T. Lawrence, Theodore S. Rosenberg, Steven A.
Contents	The Cancer Genome -- Mechanisms of Genomic Instability -- Epigenetics of Cancer -- Telomeres, Telomerase, and Cancer -- Cell Signaling Growth Factors and Their Receptors -- Cell Cycle -- Mechanisms of Cell Death -- Cancer Metabolism -- Angiogenesis -- Invasion and Metastasis -- Cancer Stem Cells -- Biology of Personalized Cancer Medicine -- Tobacco -- Cancer Susceptibility Syndromes -- DNA Viruses -- RNA Viruses -- Inflammation -- Chemical Factors -- Physical Factors -- Dietary Factors -- Obesity and Physical Activity -- Epidemiologic Methods -- Global Cancer Incidence and Mortality -- Trends in Cancer Mortality -- Surgical Oncology: General Issues -- Surgical Oncology: Laparoscopic Surgery -- Radiation Oncology -- Medical Oncology -- Assessment of Clinical Response -- Cancer Immunotherapy -- Health Services Research and Economics of Cancer Care -- Pharmacokinetics and Pharmacodynamics -- Pharmacogenomics -- Alkylating Agents -- Platinum Analogs -- Antimetabolites -- Topoisomerase-Interacting Agents -- Antimicrotubule Agents -- Targeted Therapy with Small Molecule Kinase Inhibitors -- Histone Deacetylase Inhibitors and Demethylating Agents -- Proteasome Inhibitors -- Poly(ADP-Ribose) Polymerase Inhibitors -- Miscellaneous Chemotherapeutic Agents -- Interferons -- Interleukin Therapy -- Antisense Agents -- Antiangiogenesis Agents -- Monoclonal Antibodies -- Endocrine

Manipulation -- Preventive Cancer Vaccines -- Tobacco Dependence and Its Treatment -- Role of Surgery in Cancer Prevention -- Principles of Cancer Risk Reduction Intervention -- Retinoids, Carotenoids, and Other Micronutrients in Cancer Prevention -- Drugs and Nutritional Extracts for Cancer Risk Reduction (Chemoprevention) -- Principles of Cancer Screening -- Early Detection Using Proteomics -- Screening for Gastrointestinal Cancers -- Screening for Gynecologic Cancers -- Screening for Breast Cancer -- Screening for Prostate Cancer -- Screening for Lung Cancer -- Genetic Counseling -- Vascular Access and Specialized Techniques -- Interventional Radiology -- Functional Imaging -- Molecular Imaging -- Photodynamic Therapy -- Biomarkers -- Design and Analysis of Clinical Trials -- Molecular Biology of Head and Cancers -- Treatment of Head and Neck Cancer -- Rehabilitation after Treatment of Head and Neck Cancer -- Molecular Biology of Lung Cancer -- Non-Small Cell Lung Cancer -- Small Cell and Neuroendocrine Tumors of the Lung -- Neoplasms of the Mediastinum -- Molecular Biology of the Esophagus and Stomach -- Cancer of the Esophagus -- Cancer of the Stomach -- Molecular Biology of Pancreas Cancer -- Cancer of the Pancreas -- Molecular Biology of Liver Cancer -- Cancer of the Liver -- Cancer of the Biliary Tree -- Cancer of the Small Intestine -- Gastrointestinal Stromal Tumor -- Molecular Biology of Colorectal Cancer -- Cancer of the Colon -- Cancer of the Rectum -- Cancer of the Anal Region -- Molecular Biology of Kidney Cancer -- Cancer of the Kidney -- Molecular Biology of Bladder Cancer -- Cancer of the Bladder, Ureter, and Renal Pelvis -- Molecular Biology of Prostate Cancer -- Cancer of the Prostate -- Cancer of the Urethra and Penis -- Cancer of the Testis -- Molecular Biology of Gynecologic -- Cancer of the Cervix, Vagina, and Vulva -- Cancers of the Uterine Body -- Gestational Trophoblastic Neoplasms -- Ovarian Cancer, Fallopian

Tube Carcinoma, and Peritoneal Carcinoma -- Molecular Biology of Breast Cancer -- Malignant Tumors of the Breast -- Molecular Biology of Endocrine Tumors -- Thyroid Tumors -- Parathyroid Tumors -- Adrenal Tumors -- Pancreatic Neuroendocrine Tumors -- Neuroendocrine (Carcinoid) Tumors and the Carcinoid Syndrome -- Multiple Endocrine Neoplasias -- Molecular Biology of Soft Tissue Sarcoma -- Soft Tissue Sarcoma -- Sarcomas of Bone -- Cancer of the Skin -- Molecular Biology of Cutaneous Melanoma -- Cutaneous Melanoma -- Molecular Biology of Central Nervous System Tumors -- Neoplasms of the Central Nervous System -- Molecular Biology of Childhood Cancers -- Solid Tumors of Childhood -- Leukemias and Lymphomas of Childhood -- Molecular Biology of Lymphomas -- Hodgkin Lymphoma -- Non-Hodgkin Lymphomas -- Cutaneous Lymphomas -- Primary Central Nervous System Lymphoma -- Molecular Biology of Acute Leukemias -- Management of Acute Leukemias -- Molecular Biology of Chronic Leukemias -- Chronic Myelogenous Leukemia -- Chronic Lymphocytic Leukemias -- Myelodysplastic Syndromes -- Plasma Cell Neoplasms -- Cancer of Unknown Primary Site -- Benign and Malignant Mesothelioma -- Peritoneal Surface Malignancy -- Intraocular Melanoma -- ALDS-Related Malignancies -- Transplantation-Related Malignancies -- Superior Vena Cava Syndrome -- Increased Intracranial Pressure -- Spinal Cord Compression -- Metabolic Emergencies -- Metastatic Cancer to the Brain -- Metastatic Cancer to the Lung -- Metastatic Cancer to the Liver -- Metastatic Cancer to the Bone -- Malignant Effusions of the Pleura and the Pericardium -- Malignant Ascites -- Paraneoplastic Syndromes -- Autologous Stem Cell Transplantation -- Allogeneic Stem Cell Transplantation -- Infections in the Cancer Patient -- Leukopenia and Thrombocytopenia -- Cancer-Associated Thrombosis -- Nausea and

	Vomiting -- Diarrhea and Constipation -- Oral Complications -- Pulmonary Toxicity -- Cardiac Toxicity -- Hair Loss -- Gonadal Dysfunction -- Fatigue -- Second Primary Cancers -- Neurocognitive Effects -- Cancer Survivorship -- Management of Cancer Pain -- Nutritional Support -- Sexual Problems -- Psychological Issues in Cancer -- Communicating News to the Cancer Patient -- Specialized Care of the Terminally Ill -- Community Resources -- Rehabilitation of the Cancer Patient -- Regulatory Issues -- Health Disparities in Cancer -- Cancer Information on the Internet -- Complementary, Alternative, and Integrative Therapies in Cancer Care.
Subjects	Cancer. Oncology. Neoplasms.
Notes	Includes bibliographical references and index.

Flour and breads and their fortification in health and disease prevention

LCCN	2011414005
Type of material	Book
Main title	Flour and breads and their fortification in health and disease prevention / edited by Victor R. Preedy, Ronald Ross Watson, Vinood B. Patel.
Edition	1st ed.
Published/Created	Amsterdam; Boston: Elsevier/Academic Press, 2011.
Description	xvii, 524 p.: ill.; 29 cm.
ISBN	9780123808868 (hbk.) 0123808863 (hbk.)
LC classification	TX595.F5 F57 2011
Related names	Preedy, Victor R. Watson, Ronald R. (Ronald Ross) Patel, Vinood B.
Contents	Contents of Section 1, Flours and breads: The science of doughs and bread quality -- Monitoring flour performance in bread making -- South Indian parotta: an unleavened, flat bread -- Sourdough breads -- Focaccia Italian flat fatty bread -- Flour and bread from black, purple and blue-colored wheats -- Emmer

(Triticum turgidum spp. dicoccum) flour and breads -- Einkorn (Triticum monococcum) flour and bread -- Maize: composition, bioactive constituents and unleavened bread -- Amaranth: potential source for flour enrichment -- Quinoa: protein and non protein tryptophan in comparison with other cereal and legume flours and bread -- Sorghum flour and flour products: production, nutritional quality and fortification -- Buckwheat flour and bread -- Non-starch polysaccharides in maize and oat: ferulated arabinoxylans and [beta]-glucans -- Gluten-free bread: sensory, physicochemical and nutritional aspects -- Dietary fiber from brewer's spent grain as a functional ingredient in bread making technology -- Composite flours and breads: potentials of local crops in developing countries -- Legume composite flours and baked goods: nutritional, functional, sensory and phytochemical qualities -- Potential use of okra seed (Abelmoschus esculentus Moench) flour for food fortification and effects of processing -- Apricot kernel flour and its use in maintaining health -- Macadamia flours: nutritious ingredients for baked goods -- Banana and mango flours -- Use of potato flour in bread and flat bread. Contents of Section 2, Fortification of flour and breads and their metabolic effects: Mineral fortification of whole wheat flour: an overview -- Iron particle size in iron-fortified bread -- Iodine fortification of bread: experiences from Australia and New Zealand -- Phytochemical fortification of flour and bread -- Carotenoids of sweet potato, cassava and maize and their use in bread and flour fortification -- Production and nutraceutical properties of breads fortified with DHA and omega-3 containing oils -- Fortification with free amino acids affects acrylamide content in yeast leavened bread -- Barley [beta]-glucans and fiber-rich fractions as functional ingredients in flat and pan breads -- Antioxidant activity and phenolics in breads with added barley flour -- Partial substitution of wheat flour

	with chempedak (Artocarpus integer) seed flour in bread -- Effect of starch addition to fluid dough during the bread making process -- Fermentation as a tool to improve healthy properties of bread -- Apple pomace (by-product of fruit juice industry) as a flour fortification strategy -- Use of sweet potato in bread and flour fortification -- Fortification of bread with soy proteins to normalize serum cholesterol and triacylglycerol levels -- Dietary breads and impact on postprandial parameters -- Fortification of vitamin B-12 to flour and the metabolic response -- Metabolic effects of [beta]-glucans addition to corn maize flour -- Lupine kernel fiber: metabolic effects in human intervention studies and use as supplement in wheat bread -- Metabolic effects of propionic acid-enriched breads -- Folic acid and colon cancer: impact of wheat flour fortification with folic acid -- Effects of the soybean flour diet on insulin secretion and action -- Metabolic effects of bread fortified with wheat sprouts and bioavailability of ferulic acid from wheat bran.
Subjects	Flour as food. Food additives. Enriched foods. Enriched cereal products. Bread. Medicine, Preventive. Bread. Flour. Food, Fortified. Nutritive Value.
Notes	Includes bibliographical references and index.

Food carotenoids: chemistry, biology and technology

LCCN	2015018743
Type of material	Book
Personal name	Rodriguez-Amaya, Delia B., author.
Main title	Food carotenoids: chemistry, biology and technology / Delia Rodriguez-Amaya, University of Campinas, Universidade Federal da Fronteira Sul, Brazil.

Published/Produced	Chichester, West Sussex, UK; Hoboken, NJ, USA: John Wiley and Sons, Inc., [2016] ©2016
Description	xiv, 308 pages: illustrations; 25 cm.
ISBN	9781118733301 (cloth) 1118733304
LC classification	QP671.C35 R63 2016
Contents	Nomenclature, structures, physical and chemical properties -- Biosynthesis and metabolism -- Qualitative and quantitative analysis -- In vitro assays of bioaccessibility and antioxidant capacity -- Composition and influencing factors -- Effects of processing and storage -- Isomerization and oxidation -- Carotenoids as food colorants and precursors of aroma compounds -- Bioaccessibility and bioavailability -- Provitamin A activity -- Carotenoids and chronic diseases.
Subjects	Carotenoids. Carotenoids.
Notes	Includes bibliographical references and index.
Additional formats	Online version: Rodriguez-Amaya, Delia, author. Food carotenoids Chichester, West Sussex; Hoboken, NJ: John Wiley and Sons, Inc., [2016] 9781118864333 (DLC) 2015019448
Series	IFT Press series IFT Press series.

Fortified foods with vitamins: analytical concepts to assure better and safer products

LCCN	2012472708
Type of material	Book
Main title	Fortified foods with vitamins: analytical concepts to assure better and safer products / edited by Michael Rychlik.
Published/Created	Weinheim: Wiley-VCH, c2011.
Description	xxii, 292 p.: ill.; 25 cm.
ISBN	9783527330782 (alk. paper) 352733078X (alk. paper) 9783527634170 (ePDF ISBN)

9783527634163 (ePub ISBN)
9783527634187 (Mobi)
9783527634156 (oBook ISBN)

LC classification TX553.V5 F67 2011

Related names Rychlik, Michael, Ph. D.

Contents Perspectives and General Methodology in Vitamin Analysis. Stable Isotope Dilution Assays in Vitamin Analysis-A Review of Principles and Applications / Michael Rychlik -- Analytical Methods to Assess the Bioavailability of Water-Soluble Vitamins in Food-Exemplified by Folate / Cornelia M Witthoft -- Quantitation of Vitamins Using Microbiological Assays in Microtiter Formats / Wolfgang Weber, Sabine Monch, Michael Rychlik, Sylvia Stengl -- Biosensors in Vitamin Analysis of Foods / Anthony O'Kane, Lennart Wahlstrom -- International Perspectives in Vitamin Analysis and Legislation in Vitamin Fortification / Michael Rychlik -- Analysis of Water-Soluble Vitamins. HPLC Determination of Thiamin in Fortified Foods / Roland Bitsch, Irmgard Bitsch -- HPLC Determination of Riboflavin in Fortified Foods / Roland Bitsch, Irmgard Bitsch -- HPLC-MS Determination of Vitamin C in Fortified Food Products / Antonia Garrido Frenich, Jose Luis Martinez Vidal, Remedios Fernandez Fernandez, Roberto Romero-Gonzalez -- Quantitation of Pantothenic Acid in Fortified Foods by Stable Isotope Dilution Analysis and Method Comparison with a Microbiological Assay / Michael Rychlik -- Optimization of HPLC Methods for Analyzing Added Folic Acid in Fortified Foods / Padmanaban G Krishnan, Sudheer R Musukula, Michael Rychlik, David R Nelson, Jonathan W DeVries, John L MacDonald -- Studies on New Folates in Fortified Foods and Assessment of Their Bioavailability and Bioactivity / Michael Rychlik, Dora Roth-Meier -- Analysis of Vitamin B by HPLC / Bo Chen, Da-Jin Yang -- Microbiological Detection of Vitamin B and Other Vitamins / Fumio Watanabe, Yukinori Yabuta --

	Multimethod for Water-Soluble Vitamins in Foods by Using LC-MS / Alessandra Gentili, Fulvia Caretti -- Analysis of Fat-Soluble Vitamins. Analysis of Carotenoids / Volker Bohm -- HPLC Determination of Vitamin E in Fortified Foods / Afaf Kamal-Eldin, Jelena Jastrebova -- Determination of Vitamin D by LC-MS/MS / Dorit Kern -- Quantitation of Vitamin K in Foods / Sameh Ahmed, Naoya Kishikawa, Kaname Ohyama, Naotaka Kuroda -- Trace Analysis of Carotenoids and Fat-Soluble Vitamins in Some Food Matrices by LC-APCI-MS/MS / Alessandra Gentili, Fulvia Caretti.
Subjects	Food--Vitamin content. Enriched foods.
Notes	Includes bibliographical references and index.

Fruit and cereal bioactives: sources, chemistry, and applications

LCCN	2010044816
Type of material	Book
Main title	Fruit and cereal bioactives: sources, chemistry, and applications / edited by Özlem Tokuşoğlu, Clifford Hall III.
Published/Created	Boca Raton, [Fla.]: CRC Press, c2011.
Description	xiv, 459 p. [8] p. of plates: ill. (some col.); 26 cm.
ISBN	9781439806654 (hardcover: alkaline paper)
LC classification	QK865 .F78 2011
Related names	Tokuşoğlu, Özlem, editor. Hall, Clifford, III, editor.
Summary	"Presenting up-to-date data in an easy-to-use format, this comprehensive overview of the chemistry of bioactive components of fruits and cereals addresses the role of these compounds in determining taste, flavor, and color, as well as recent claims of anticarginogenic, antimutagenic, and antioxidant capabilities. It provides detailed information on both beneficial bioactives such as phenolics, flavonoids, tocols, carotenoids, phytosterols, and avenanthramides and toxicant compounds including mycotoxins; aflatoxins, ocratoxin A, patulin, citrinin, cyclopiazonic

	acid, fumonisin, and zearalenon. A valuable resource for current knowledge and further research, it offers critical reviews, recent research, case studies, and references" --Provided by publisher.
Subjects	Fruit--Composition. Grain--Composition. Phytochemicals--Physiological effect. Fruit--chemistry. Cereals--chemistry. Dietary Supplements. Phytotherapy. Plant Extracts--therapeutic use.
Notes	Includes bibliographical references and index.

Fruit and vegetable phytochemicals: chemistry, nutritional value and stability

LCCN	2009031846
Type of material	Book
Main title	Fruit and vegetable phytochemicals: chemistry, nutritional value and stability / [editors]: Laura A. de la Rosa, Emilio Alvarez-Parrilla, Gustavo A. González-Aguilar.
Published/Created	Ames, Iowa: Wiley-Blackwell, 2010.
Description	xi, 367 p.: ill.; 26 cm.
ISBN	9780813803203 (hardback)
LC classification	QK898.P764 F78 2010
Related names	Rosa, Laura A. de la. Alvarez-Parrilla, Emilio. González-Aguilar, Gustavo A.
Subjects	Phytochemicals. Polyphenols. Carotenoids. Fruit--Analysis. Vegetables--Analysis.
Notes	Includes bibliographical references and index.

Frying of food: oxidation, nutrient and non-nutrient antioxidants, biologically active compounds and high temperatures, second edition

LCCN	2010043667
Type of material	Book
Main title	Frying of food: oxidation, nutrient and non-nutrient antioxidants, biologically active compounds and high temperatures, second edition / [edited by] Dimitrios Boskou, Ibrahim Elmadfa.
Edition	2nd ed.
Published/Created	Boca Raton: CRC Press, c2011.
Description	x, 318 p.: ill.; 24 cm.
ISBN	9781439806821 (hardback)
LC classification	TP670. F79 2011
Related names	Boskou, Dimitrios. Elmadfa, I.
Summary	"*Frying of Food* is the first reference to examine frying of food from the point of view of changes occurring to biologically-active constituents and the effects of such changes on the stability, performance and nutritive value of frying oil. It focuses on the nature of the frying media and discusses changes to non-glyceride components, especially nutritive and non-utritive antioxidants. This important resource concentrates mainly on two factors that influence the deterioration of a fat at elevated temperatures: the nature of the heated fat and the presence of oxidation retardants, especially those naturally occurring in oils or obtained from natural sources. Discussions include important biologically active ingredients present in oils and fats (such as antioxidant vitamins and carotenoids) and minor constituents (such as phytosterols, phospholipids and hydrocarbons), which appear to affect the performance of a heated oil and/or may also be categorized as functional. *Frying of Food* also discusses olar phenolic compounds, which have an impact on the stability of oils at high temperatures. Food and lipid chemists, food technologists and product developers involved in the processing of foods

by frying, and to those involved in fat and oil research, in quality assessment of heated fats, and in improving dietary fat intake profiles will find this book valuable"-- Provided by publisher.
"This important resource concentrates mainly on two factors that influence the deterioration of a fat at elevated temperatures: the nature of the heated fat and the presence of oxidation retardants, especially those naturally occurring in oils or obtained from natural sources. Discussions include important biologically active ingredients present in oils and fats and minor constituents, which appear to affect the performance of a heated oil and/or may also be categorized as functional. Frying of Food also discusses olar phenolic compounds, which have an impact on the stability of oils at high temperatures"-- Provided by publisher.

Subjects	Oils and fats, Edible--Effect of temperature on. Frying. Technology & Engineering / Food Science
Notes	Includes bibliographical references and index.

Functional foods and nutraceuticals

LCCN	2012937216
Type of material	Book
Personal name	Aluko, Rotimi E.
Main title	Functional foods and nutraceuticals / Rotimi E. Aluko.
Published/Created	New York, NY: Springer, c2012.
Description	xii, 155 p: ill.; 27 cm.
ISBN	9781461434795 (alk. paper) 1461434793 (alk. paper) 9781461434801 (e-ISBN) 1461434807 (e-ISBN)
LC classification	QP144.F85 A48 2012
Contents	Part 1. Nutrient Components of Foods -- Bioactive Carbohydrates -- Bioactive Lipids -- Bioactive Peptides -- Bioactive Polyphenols and Carotenoids -- Part 2. Specific Functional Foods -- Soybean -- Fruits and Vegetables -- Milk and Milk Products -- Fish -- Miscellaneous Foods and Food Components.

Subjects	Functional foods. Functional Food. Dietary Supplements. Nutritive Value.
Notes	Includes bibliographical references and index.
Series	Food science text series, 1572-0330 Food science text series.

Microbial carotenoids from bacteria and microalgae: Methods and protocols

LCCN	2012937073
Type of material	Book
Main title	Microbial carotenoids from bacteria and microalgae: methods and protocols / edited by José-Luis Barredo.
Published/Created	New York: Humana Press, c2012.
Description	xi, 355 p.: ill.; 27 cm.
ISBN	9781617798788 (alk. paper) 1617798789 (alk. paper) 9781617798795 (e-ISBN) 1617798797 (e-ISBN)
LC classification	QP671.C35 M53 2012
Related names	Barredo, José-Luis.
Contents	Pathways of carotenoid biosynthesis in bacteria and microalgae / J. Paniagua-Michel, Jorge Olmos-Soto, and Manuel Acosta Ruiz -- Selection and taxonomic identification of carotenoid-producing marine actinomycetes / Francisco Romero -- Isolation, characterization, and diversity of novel radiotolerant carotenoid-producing bacteria / Dalal Asker ... [et al.] -- Novel radio-tolerant astaxanthin-producing bacterium reveals a new astaxanthin derivative: astaxanthin dirhamnoside / Dalal Asker ... [et al.] -- Novel zeaxanthin-producing bacteria isolated from a radioactive hot spring water / Dalal Asker ... [et al.] -- Novel approach in the biosynthesis of functional carotenoids in Escherichia coli / Hisashi Harada and Norihiko Misawa -- Engineering Escherichia coli for canthaxanthin and ataxanthin biosynthesis / Qiong Cheng and Luan Tao -- Analysis of canthaxanthin

production by Gordonia jacobaea / Patricia Veiga-Crespo ... [et al.] -- Isolation and light-stimulated expression of canthaxanthin and spirilloxanthin biosynthesis genes from the photosynthetic bacterium Bradyrhizobium sp. Strain ORS278 / Eric Giraud and Andre Vermeglio -- Construction of carotenoid biosynthetic pathways through chromosomal integration in methane-utilizing bacterium Methylomonas sp. strain 16a / Rick W. Ye and Kristen Kelly -- Genetic modification in Bacillus subtilis for production of C30 carotenoids / Isamu Maeda -- Carotenoids' production from halophilic bacteria / Maria de Lourdes Moreno ... [et al.] -- Construction and utilization of carotenoid reporter systems: identification of chromosomal integration sites that support suitable expression of biosynthetic genes and pathways / Pamela L. Sharpe and Deana J. DiCosimo -- Directed evolution of carotenoid synthases for the production of unnatural carotenoids / Maiko Furubayashi and Daisuke Umeno -- High-Throughput Screen for the Identi fi cation of improved catalytic activity: b-carotene hydroxylase / Mark A. Scaife ... [et al.] -- DNA fingerprinting intron-sizing method to accomplish a specific, rapid, and sensitive identification of carotenogenic Dunaliella species / Jorge Olmos-Soto ... [et al.] -- Ketocarotenoid biosynthesis in transgenic microalgae expressing a foreign beta-C-4-carotene oxygenase gene / Marta Vila ... [et al.] -- Characterization of carotenogenesis genes in the cyanobacterium Anabaena sp. PCC 7120 / Hajime Masukawa, Mari Mochimaru, and Shinichi Takaichi -- Obtaining lutein-rich extract from microalgal biomass at preparative scale / Jose M. Fernandez-Sevilla, F. Gabriel Acien Fernandez, and Emilio Molina Grima -- NMR-based isotopologue profiling of microbial carotenoids / Eva Eylert, Adelbert Bacher, and Wolfgang Eisenreich -- Analysis of diapocarotenoids found in pigmented Bacillus species / Laura Perez-Fons and Paul D. Fraser.

Subjects	Carotenoids--Laboratory manuals. Carotenoids--biosynthesis--Laboratory Manuals. Bacteria--chemistry--Laboratory Manuals. Microalgae--chemistry--Laboratory Manuals.
Notes	Includes bibliographical references and index.
Series	Methods in molecular biology, 1064-3745; 892 Methods in molecular biology (Clifton, N.J.); v. 892. 1064-3745

Microbial carotenoids from fungi: methods and protocols

LCCN	2012939488
Type of material	Book
Main title	Microbial carotenoids from fungi: methods and protocols / edited by José-Luis Barredo.
Published/Created	New York: Humana Press, c2012.
Description	xi, 290 p.: ill. (some col.); 27 cm.
ISBN	9781617799174 (hbk.: alk. paper) 1617799173 (hbk.: alk. paper) 9781617799181 (ebk.)
LC classification	QK898.C34 M53 2012
Related names	Barredo, José-Luis.
Contents	Metabolic engineering of Mucor circinelloides for zeaxanthin production / Marta Rodríguez-Sáiz, Juan-Luis de la Fuente, and José-Luis Barredo -- Bioengineering of oleaginous yeast Yarrowia lipolytica for lycopene production / Rick W. Ye, Pamela L. Sharpe, and Quinn Zhu -- Peroxisome targeting of lycopene pathway enzymes in Pichia pastoris / Pyung Cheon Lee -- Production, extraction, and quantification of astaxanthin by Xanthophyllomyces dendrorhous or Haematococcus pluvialis: standardized techniques / Alma Rosa Domínguez-Bocanegra -- Isolation and selection of new astaxanthin producing strains of Xanthophyllomyces dendrorhous / Diego Libkind, Martín Moliné, and Celia Tognetti -- Isolation and characterization of extrachromosomal double-stranded RNA elements in Xanthophyllomyces dendrorhous / Marcelo Baeza, María Fernández-Lobato, and Víctor

	Cifuentes
Subjects	Carotenoids.
	Fungal molecular biology.
	Carotenoids--biosynthesis--Laboratory Manuals.
	Fungi--Laboratory Manuals.
	Biotechnology--methods--Laboratory Manuals.
Notes	Includes bibliographical references and index.
Series	Methods in molecular biology, 1940-6029; 898
	Springer protocols
	Methods in molecular biology (Clifton, N.J.); 898.
	Springer protocols.

Microbial metabolic engineering: methods and protocols

LCCN	2011943294
Type of material	Book
Main title	Microbial metabolic engineering: methods and protocols / edited by Qiong Cheng.
Published/Created	New York, NY: Humana Press, c2012.
Description	xii, 319 p.: ill. (some col.); 27 cm.
ISBN	9781617794827 (alk. paper)
	1617794821 (alk. paper)
	9781617794834 (e-ISBN)
	161779483X (e-ISBN)
LC classification	QR88 .M526 2012
Related names	Cheng, Qiong.
Contents	Screening for cellulases with industrial value and their use in biomass conversion / Julia Jüergensen, Nele Ilmberger, and Wolfgang R. Streit -- Reversal of NAD(P)H cofactor dependence by protein engineering / Sabinc Bastian and Frances H. Arnold -- Quantifying plasmid copy number to investigate plasmid dosage effects associated with directed protein evolution / Samuel Million-Weaver ... [et al.] -- High isoprenoid flux Escherichia coli as a host for carotenoids production / Wonchul Suh -- Mutagenic inverted repeats assisted genome engineering (MIRAGE) in Saccharomyces cerevisiae: deletion of gal7 / Nikhil U. Nair and Huimin Zhao -- Creation of new metabolic pathways or improvement of existing metabolic

enzymes by in vivo evolution in Escherichia coli / Isabelle Meynial-Salles and Philippe Soucaille -- Bioluminescent reporter genes for promoter discovery / Tina K. Van Dyk -- Recombination-based DNA assembly and mutagenesis methods for metabolic engineering / Xiquan Liang ... [et al.] -- Ethanol-tolerant gene identification in Clostridium thermocellum using pyro-resequencing for metabolic engineering / Shihui Yang, Dawn M. Klingeman, and Steven D. Brown -- Use of proteomic tools in microbial engineering for biofuel production / Shaoming Mao ... [et al.] -- Metabolic engineering of antibiotic-producing Actinomycetes using in vitro transposon mutagenesis / Andrew R. Reeves and J. Mark Weber -- Use FACS sorting in metabolic engineering of Escherichia coli for increased peptide production / Qiong Cheng ... [et al.] -- Using flux balance analysis to guide microbial metabolic engineering / Kathleen A. Curran, Nathan C. Crook, and Hal S. Alper -- Using an advanced microfermentor system for strain screening and fermentation optimization / Dongming Xie -- Rapid strain evaluation using dynamic DO-stat fed-batch fermentation under scale-down conditions / Jun Sun -- Preparation and evaluation of lignocellulosic biomass hydrolysates for growth by ethanologenic yeasts / Ying Zha ... [et al.] -- Engineering whole-cell biosensors with no antibiotic markers for monitoring aromatic compounds in the environment / Aitor de las Heras and Víctor de Lorenzo -- Metabolic engineering for acetate control in large scale fermentation / Yong Tao, Qiong Cheng, and Alexander D. Kopatsis -- Minimization and prevention of phage infections in bioprocesses / Marcin Los.

Subjects Microbial metabolism--Laboratory manuals.
Microbial genetics--Laboratory manuals.
Genetics, Microbial--Laboratory Manuals.
Bioengineering--Laboratory Manuals.

Notes Includes bibliographical references and index.

Series	Methods in molecular biology, 1064-3745; 834 Springer protocols Methods in molecular biology (Clifton, N.J.); v. 834. Springer protocols.

Microbiology for dummies

LCCN	2014936394
Type of material	Book
Personal name	Stearns, Jennifer C.
Main title	Microbiology for dummies / Jennifer C. Stearns, Julie Kaiser, and Michael G. Surette.
Published/Produced	Hoboken: For Dummies, a Wiley brand, [2015]
Description	xii, 366 pages: illustrations; 24 cm.
ISBN	9781118871188 (pbk.) 1118871189 (pbk.)
LC classification	QR56 .S83 2015
Related names	Kaiser, Julie. Surette, Michael G.
Summary	Does microbiology make your head spin? The authors make the subject accessible and fun, to help you grasp life at the cellular level. Whether you need to score big at exam time, or just want to satisfy your curiosity, this guide will help you discover the main types of microorganisms and the benefits of their microbial communities.-- Source other than Library of Congress.
Contents	pt. I. Getting started with microbiology -- 1. Microbiology and you -- Why microbiology? -- Introducing microorganisms -- Deconstructing microbiology -- 2. Microbiology: the young science -- Before microbiology: misconceptions and superstitions -- Discovering microorganisms -- Debunking the myth of spontaneous generation -- Improving medicine, from surgery to antibiotics and more -- Looking at microbiology outside the human body -- The future of microbiology -- Frontiers -- Challenges -- 3. Microbes: they're everywhere and the can do everything -- Habitat diversity -- Metabolic diversity -- Getting energy -- Capturing carbon -- Making enzymes -- Secondary metabolism -- The intersection of microbes

and everyone else -- pt. II. Balancing the dynamics of microbial life -- Seeing the shapes of cells -- Life on a minute scale: considering the size of prokaryotes -- The cell: an overview -- Scaling the outer membrane and cell walls -- Examining the outer membrane -- Exploring the cell wall -- Other important cell structures -- Divining cell division -- Tackling transport systems -- Passive transport -- Active transport -- Keeping things clean with efflux pumps -- Getting around with locomotion -- 5. Making sense of metabolism -- Converting with enzymes -- In charge of energy: oxidation and reduction -- Donating and accepting electrons -- Bargaining with energy-rich compounds -- Storing energy for later -- Breaking down catabolism -- Digesting glycolysis -- Stepping along with respiration and electron carriers -- Moving with the proton motive force -- Turning the citric acid cycle -- Stacking up with anabolism -- Creating amino acids and nucleic acids -- Making sugars and polysaccharides -- Putting together fatty acids and lipids -- 6. Getting the gist of microbial genetics -- Organizing genetic material -- DNA: the recipe for life -- Perfect plasmids -- DNA replication -- Assembling the cellular machinery -- Making messenger RNA -- Other types of RNA -- synthesizing protein -- DNA regulation -- Regulating protein function -- Changing the genetic code -- Slight adjustments -- Major rearrangements -- 7. Measuring microbial growth -- Getting growth requirements right -- Physical requirements -- Chemical requirements -- Culturing microbes in the lab -- Observing microbes -- Counting small things -- Seeing morphology -- Calculating cell division and population growth -- dividing cells -- Following growth phases -- Inhibiting microbial growth -- Physical methods -- Disinfectants -- pt. III. Sorting out microbial diversity -- 8. Appreciating microbial ancestry -- Where did microbes come from? -- Tracing the origins of life -- Diversifying early prokaryotes -- The impact of prokaryotes on the early earth -- Hitching a ride: endosymbiosis -- Understanding evolution -- Studying evolution -- Choosing marker genes -- Seeing the direction of gene transfer in prokaryotes -- Classifying and naming microbes -- Climbing the tree of life -- 9. Harnessing energy, fixing carbon -- Forging ahead with autotrophic processes -- Fixing carbon -- Using the energy in light -- Harvesting light: chlorophylls and bacteriochlorophylls -- Helping photosynthesis out: carotenoids and phycobilins -- Generating oxygen (or not): oxygenic and anoxygenic photosynthesis -- Getting energy from the elements: chemolithotrophy -- Harnessing hydrogen -- Securing electrons from sulfur -- Pumping iron -- Oxidizing nitrate and ammonia -- 10. comparing respiration and fermentation -- Lifestyles of the rich and facultative -- Digging into respiration -- Spinning the citric acid cycle -- Stepping down the electron transport chain -- Respiring anaerobically -- Figuring out fermentation -- 11. Uncovering a variety of habitats -- Defining a habitat -- Understanding nutrient cycles -- Carbon cycling -- Nitrogen cycling -- Sulfur cycling -- Phosphorous cycles in the ocean -- Microbes socializing in communities -- Using quorum sensing to communication -- Living in biofilms -- Exploring microbial mats -- Discovering microbes in aquatic and terrestrial habitats -- Thriving in water -- Swarming soils -- Getting along with plants and animals -- Living with plants -- Living with animals -- Living with insects -- Living with ocean creatures -- Tolerating extreme locations -- Detecting microbes in unexpected places -- pt. IV. Meeting the microbes -- 12. Meet the prokaryotes -- Getting to know the bacteria -- The gram-negative bacteria: proteobacteria -- More gram-negative bacteria -- The gram-positive bacteria -- Acquainting yourself with the archaea -- Scalding: extreme thermophiles -- Acidic: extreme acidophiles -- Salty: extreme halophiles -- Not terribly extreme archaea -- 13. Say hello to eukaryotes -- Fun with fungi -- Figuring out fungal physiology -- Itemizing fungal diversity -- Interacting with plant roots -- Ascomycetes -- MUshrooms: basidiomycetes -- Perusing the protists -- Making us sick: apicoplexans -- Making plants sick: oomycetes -- chasing amoeba and ciliates -- Encountering the algae -- 14. Examining the vastness of viruses -- Hijacking cells -- Frugal viral structure -- Simplifying viral function -- Making heads or tails of bacteriophage -- Lytic phage -- Temperate phage -- Transposable phage -- Discussing viruses of eukaryotes -- Infecting animal cells -- Following plant viruses -- How host cells fight back -- Restriction enzymes -- CRISPR -- Interfering with RNA viruses: RNAi -- pt. V. Seeing the impact of microbes -- 15. Understanding microbes in human health and disease -- Clarifying the host immune response -- Putting up barriers to infection -- Inflammation -- Innate immunity -- Adaptive immunity -- Antibodies -- Relying on antimicrobials for treating disease -- Fundamental features of antibiotics -- Targets of destruction -- Unraveling microbial drug resistance -- Discovering new antibiotics -- Searching out superbugs -- Vancomycin-resistant enterococci -- Methicillin-resistant staphylococcus aureus -- Clostridium difficile -- Extended-spectrum beta-lactamases -- Prebiotics and probiotics -- Antiviral drugs -- 16. Putting microbes to work: biotechnology -- Using recombinant DNA technology -- Making the insert -- Employing plasmids -- Restriction enzymes -- Getting microbes to take up DNA -- Using promoters to drive expression -- Expression vectors -- Folding proteins -- Metabolic load -- Long, multigene constructs -- Providing therapies -- Improving antibiotics -- Developing vaccines -- Using microbes industrially -- Protecting plants wit microbial insecticides -- Making biofuels -- Bioleaching metals -- Cleaning up with microbes -- 17. Fighting microbial diseases -- Protecting public health: epidemiology -- Tracking diseases -- Investigating outbreaks --

Identifying a microbial pathogen -- characterizing morphology -- Using biochemical tests -- Typing strains with phage -- Using serology -- Testing antibiotic susceptibility -- Understanding vaccines -- How vaccines work -- Ranking the types of vaccines -- pt. VI. New frontiers in microbiology -- 18. Teasing apart communities -- Studying microbial communities -- Borrowing from ecology -- Seeing what sets microbial communities apart from plants and animals -- Observing communities: microbial ecology methods -- Selecting something special with enrichment -- Seeing cells through lenses -- Measuring microbial activity -- Identifying species using marker genes -- Getting the hang of microbial genetics and systematics -- Sequencing whole genomes -- Using metagenomics to study microbial communities -- Reading microbial transcriptomics -- Figuring out proteomics and metabolomics -- Looking for microbial dark matter -- 19. Synthesizing life -- Regulating genes: the lac operon -- Using a good natural system -- Improving a good system -- Designing genetic networks -- Switching from one state to another -- Oscillating between states -- Keeping signals short -- The synthetic biologist's toolbox -- Making it modular -- Participating in iGEM competition -- pt. VII. The part of tens -- 20. Ten (or so) diseases caused by microbes -- Ebola -- Anthrax -- Influenza -- Tuberculosis -- HIV -- Cholera -- Smallpox -- Primary amoebic menigoencephalitis -- The unknown -- 21. Ten great uses for microbes -- Making delicious foods -- Growing legumes -- Brewing beer, liquor, and wine -- Killing insect pests -- Treating sewage -- Contributing to medicine -- Setting up your aquarium -- Making and breaking down biodegradable plastics -- Turning over compostable waste -- Maintaining a balance -- 22. Ten great uses for microbiology -- Medical care -- Dental care -- Veterinary care -- Monitoring the environment -- Making plants happy -- Keeping fish swimming strong -- Producing food, wine, and beer -- Science

	hacking -- Looking for microbes in clean rooms -- Producing pharmaceuticals.
Subjects	Microbiology--Popular works. Microbiological Phenomena. Communicable Diseases--microbiology. Immunity. Microbiology.
Form/Genre	Popular works.
Notes	Includes index.
Series	--For dummies --For dummies.

Photosynthesis: plastid biology, energy conversion and carbon assimilation

LCCN	2011939834
Type of material	Book
Main title	Photosynthesis: plastid biology, energy conversion and carbon assimilation / edited by Julian J. Eaton-Rye, Baishnab C. Tripathy, and Thomas D. Sharkey.
Published/Created	Dordrecht; New York: Springer, ©2012.
Description	xxxvi, 856 pages: illustrations (some color), portraits (some color); 27 cm.
Links	Publisher description http://www.loc.gov/catdir/enhancements/fy1316/2011939834-d.html Table of contents only http://www.loc.gov/catdir/enhancements/fy1316/2011939834-t.html
ISBN	9789400715783 9400715781
LC classification	QK882 .P5387 2012
Portion of title	Plastid biology, energy conversion and carbon assimilation
Related names	Eaton-Rye, Julian J., editor of compilation. Tripathy, Baishnab C., editor of compilation. Sharkey, Thomas D., 1953- editor of compilation. Govindjee, 1932- editor of compilation.
Contents	1. The photosynthetic world / Martin F. Hohmann-Marriott and Robert E. Blankenship -- 2. Origin, evolution and division of plastids / Denis Falconet -- 3. Chlorophyll biosynthesis in higher plants / Baishnab

C. Tripathy and Gopal K. Pattanayak -- 4. Biosynthesis, localization and concentration of carotenoids in plants and algae / Hartmut K. Lichtenthaler -- 5. Assembly of light harvesting pigment-protein complexes in photosynthetic eukaryotes / Tomas Morosinotto and Roberto Bassi -- 6. Chlorophyll-binding proteins of higher plants and cyanobacteria / Roberta Croce -- 7. Plant proteomics and photosynthesis / Klaas J. van Wijk -- 8. Intracellular signaling from plastids to the nucleus / Wolfhart Rüdiger and Ulrike Oster -- 9. Role of the envelope membranes in chloroplast glycerolipid biosynthesis / Maryse A. Block, Juliette Jouhet, Eric Maréchal, Olivier Bastien, and Jacques Joyard -- 10. Leaf senescence and transformation of chloroplasts to gerontoplasts / Basanti Biswal, Pranab K. Mohaptra, Udaya C. Biswal, and Mukesh K. Raval -- 11. The role of membrane structure in acclimation to low-temperature stress / Balázs Szalontai, Illdikó domonkos, and Zoltán Gombos -- 12. Heat stress: susceptibility, recovery and regulation / Prasanna Mohanty, Vladimir D. Kreslavski, Vyacheslav V. Klimov, Dmitry A. Los, Mamoru Mimuro, Robert Carpentier, and Suleyman I. Allakhverdiev -- 13. Photosynthetic responses of plants to excess light: mechanisms and conditions for photoinhibition, excess energy dissipation and repair / Yagut Allahverdiyeva and Eva-Mari Aro -- 14. Light stress proteins in viruses, cyanobacteria and photosynthetic eukaryota / Mounia Heddad, Johannes Engelken, and Iwona Adamska -- 15. Environmentally-induced oxidative stress and its signaling / Antoine Danon -- 16. The characteristics of specific chlorophylls and their roles in biogenesis of the photosynthetic apparatus / J. Kenneth Hoober -- 17. Photosynthetic water splitting: apparatus and mechanism / Gernot Renger -- 18. Fluorescence emission from the photosynthetic apparatus / George C. Papageorgiou -- 19. Thermoluminescence / Prafullachandra Vishnu Sane,

Alexander G. Ivanov, Gunnar Öquist, and Norman P.A. Hüner -- 20. Regulation of photosystem II electron transport by bicarbonate / Iain L. McConnell, Julian J. Eaton-Rye, and Jack J.S. van Rensen -- 21. Cytochrome b_6f complex at the heart of energy transduction and redox signaling / Toivo Kallas -- 22. Energy transduction by the two molecular motors of the F_1F_0 ATP synthase / David Spetzler, Robert Ishmukhametov, Tassilo Hornung, James Martin, Justin York, Lixia Jin-Day, and Wayne D. Frasch -- 23. Electron transport in leaves: a physiological perspective / Gabriel Cornic and Neil R. Baker -- 24. Towards artificial photosynthesis / Wah Soon Chow -- 25. The uptake of CO_2 by cyanobacteria and microalgae / Hideya Fukuzawa, Teruo Ogawa, and Aaron Kaplan -- 26. Autotrophic carbon dioxide fixation / Thomas D. Sharkey and Sean E. Weise -- 27. Photosynthetic sucrose biosynthesis: an evolutionary perspective / Elspeth MacRae and John E. Lunn -- 28. Sucrose transport in higher plants: from source to sink / Naohiro Aoki, Tatsuro Hirose, and Robert T. Furbank -- 29. Photosynthesis in a CO_2-rich atmosphere / Andrew D.B. Leakey, Elizabeth A. Ainsworth, Carl J. Bernacchi, Xinguang Zhu, Stephen P. Long, and Donald R. Ort -- 30. Early pioneers of photosyntheis research / Jane F. Hill -- 31. Contributions of Govindjee, 1955-1969 / George C. Papageorgiou -- 32. Contributions of Govindjee, 1970-1999 / Julian J. Eaton-Rye -- 33. Contributions of Govindjee, 2000-2011 / Robert MacDonald Clegg.

Subjects	Photosynthesis.
Notes	Dedicated to Govindjee.
	Includes bibliographical references and index.
Series	Advances in photosynthesis and respiration; v. 34
	Advances in photosynthesis and respiration; v. 34.

Phytoplankton pigments: characterization, chemotaxonomy, and applications in oceanography

LCCN	2011009229
Type of material	Book
Main title	Phytoplankton pigments: characterization, chemotaxonomy, and applications in oceanography / edited by Suzanne Roy... [et al.].
Published/Created	Cambridge; New York: Cambridge University Press, 2011.
Description	xxvii, 845 p.: ill.; 26 cm.
Links	Cover image http://assets.cambridge.org/ 97811070/00667/cover/9781107000667.jpg
ISBN	9781107000667 (hardback)
LC classification	QK933 .P496 2011
Related names	Roy, Suzanne, 1955-
Summary	"Pigments act as tracers to elucidate the fate of phytoplankton in the world's oceans and are often associated with important biogeochemical cycles related to carbon dynamics in the oceans. They are increasingly used in in situ and remote-sensing applications, detecting algal biomass and major taxa through changes in water colour. This book is a follow-up to the 1997 volume Phytoplankton Pigments in Oceanography (UNESCO Press). Since then, there have been many advances concerning phytoplankton pigments. This book includes recent discoveries on several new algal classes particularly for the picoplankton, and on new pigments. It also includes many advances in methodologies, including liquid chromatography-mass spectrometry (LC-MS) and developments and updates on the mathematical methods used to exploit pigment information and extract the composition of phytoplankton communities. The book is invaluable primarily as a reference for students, researchers and professionals in aquatic science, biogeochemistry and remote sensing"-- Provided by publisher.
Contents	Machine generated contents note: List of contributors; Preface; Acknowledgements; List of symbols; Part I.

Chlorophylls and Carotenoids: 1. Microalgal classes and their signature pigments S. W. Jeffrey, S. W. Wright and M. Zapata; 2. Recent advances in chlorophyll and bacteriochlorophyll biosynthesis R. J. Porra, U. Oster and H. Scheer; 3. Carotenoid metabolism in phytoplankton M. Lohr; Part II. Methodology Guidance: 4. New HPLC separation techniques J. L. Garrido, R. L. Airs, F. Rodri;guez, L. Van Heukelem and M. Zapata; 5. The importance of a quality assurance plan for method validation and minimizing uncertainties in the HPLC analysis of phytoplankton pigments L. Van Heukelem and S. B. Hooker; Appendix: a symbology and vocabulary for an HPLC lexicon S. B. Hooker and L. Van Heukelem; 6. Quantitative interpretation of chemotaxonomic pigment data H. W. Higgins, S. W. Wright and L. Schlüter; 7. Liquid chromatography-mass spectrometry for pigment analysis R. L. Airs and J. L. Garrido; 8. Multivariate analysis of extracted pigments using spectrophotometric and spectrofluorometric methods J. Neveux, J. Seppa;la; and Y. Dandonneau; Appendix: a proven simultaneous equation assay for chlorophylls a and b using aqueous acetone and similar assays for recalcitrant algae R. J. Porra; Part III. Water-Soluble 'Pigments': 9. Phycobiliproteins K.-H. Zhao, R. J. Porra and H. Scheer; 10. UV-absorbing 'pigments': mycosporine-like amino acids J. I. Carreto, S. Roy, K. Whitehead, C. Llewellyn and M. O. Carignan; Part IV. Selected Pigment Applications in Oceanography: 11. Pigments and photoacclimation processes C. Brunet, G. Johnsen, J. Lavaud and S. Roy; 12. Pigment-based measurements of phytoplankton rates A. Guttierez-Rodriguez and M. Latasa; 13. In vivo bio-optical properties of phytoplankton pigments G. Johnsen, A. Bricaud, N. Nelson, B. B. Pre;zelin and R. R. Bidigare; 14. Optical monitoring of phytoplankton bloom pigment signatures G. Johnsen, M. A. Moline, L. H. Pettersson, J. L. Pinckney, D. V. Pozdnyakov, E. S. Egeland and O. M. Schofield; Appendix: harmful

	algae toxins and pigments E. S. Egeland; Part V. Future Perspectives: 15. Perspectives on future directions C. Llewellyn, S. Roy, G. Johnsen, E. S. Egeland, M. Chauton, G. Hallegraeff, M. Lohr, U. Oster, R. J. Porra, H. Scheer and K.-H. Zhao; Part VI. Aids for Practical Laboratory Work: Appendix A. Update on filtration, storage and extraction solvents J. L. Pinckney, D. F. Millie and L. Van Heukelem; Appendix B. The pigment analyst's guide to HPLC hardware A. R. Neeley, C. S. Thomas, S. B. Hooker and L. Van Heukelem; Appendix C. Minimum identification criteria for identifying phytoplankton pigments E. S. Egeland; Appendix D. Phytoplankton cultures for standard pigments and their suppliers S. Roy, S. W. Wright and S. W. Jeffrey; Appendix E. Commercial suppliers of phytoplankton pigments E. S. Egeland and L. Schlüter; Part VII: Phytoplankton pigments data sheets E. S. Egeland; Index.
Subjects	Phytoplankton--Composition. Phytoplankton--Chemotaxonomy. Photosynthetic pigments. Algae--Classification. Oceanography--Methodology. Science / Earth Sciences / Oceanography
Notes	Includes bibliographical references and index.
Series	Cambridge environmental chemistry series

Pigments in fruits and vegetables: genomics and dietetics

LCCN	2015933509
Type of material	Book
Main title	Pigments in fruits and vegetables: genomics and dietetics / Chunxian Chen, editor.
Published/Produced	New York: Springer, [2015] ©2015
Description	x, 277 pages: illustrations (soem color); 24 cm
ISBN	9781493923557 (hbk: acid-free paper) 1493923552 (hbk: acid-free paper) eBook
LC classification	QK898.P7 P54 2015

Related names	Chen, Chunxian, editor.
Summary	This comprehensive treatise provides insight into pigment biosynthesis and dietetics. The text includes current reviews on the genomics of carotenoid, flavonoid, and betalain biosynthesis in plants and the dietetics of these pigments in humans. Pigments biosynthesized in plants are a source of attractive colors in nature and essential nutrients in our daily fruit, vegetable, and grain diet. Deciphered from general perspectives and specific fruits and vegetables, genomics focuses on enzymatic genes and regulatory molecular mechanisms in the biosynthesis pathways to produce these pigments in plants. Dietetics focuses on the nutritional and medical benefits to human health from these pigments as nutrients, nutraceuticals, and disease prevention agents when they are ingested from pigment-abundant plant food and metabolized in human body. This work contributes to an expanding awareness of the dietetic benefits to the daily consumption of pigment-rich fruit, vegetable, and grain food.-- Source other than the Library of Congress.
Contents	Overview of Plant Pigments -- Carotenoids Biosynthesis Genomics -- Carotenoids in Human Nutrition -- Differential Transcription Factor Networks Orchestrate Flavonoid Biosynthesis -- Flavonoids Dietetics: Mechanisms and Emerging Roles of Plant Nutraceuticals -- The Betalain Secondary Metabolic Network -- Indicaxanthin Dietetics: Past, Present and Future -- Pigments in Citrus -- Pigments in Grape -- Pigments in Strawberry -- Carotenoids in Carrot -- Carotenoids in Green Vegetables and Health Aspects -- Anthocyanins in Staple Crops.
Subjects	Plant pigments.
	Biosynthesis.
	Dietetics.
Notes	Includes bibliographical references and index.

Plant isoprenoids: methods and protocols

LCCN	2014936605
Type of material	Book
Main title	Plant isoprenoids: methods and protocols / edited by Manuel Rodríguez-Concepción, Center for Research in Agricultural Genomics (CRAG), CSIC-IRTA-UAB-UB, Barcelona, Spain.
Published/Produced	New York: Humana Press, [2014] ©2014
Description	xi, 303 pages: illustrations (some color); 26 cm.
Links	Table of contents http://www.loc.gov/catdir/enhancements/fy1407/2014936605-t.html
ISBN	9781493906055 (alk. paper) 1493906054 (alk. paper)
LC classification	QK898.I76 P58 2014
Related names	Rodríguez-Concepción, Manuel, editor. Springer Science+Business Media, copyright holder.
Contents	Plant isoprenoids: A General Overview -- Measuring the Activity of 1-Deoxy-D-Xylulose 5-Phosphate Synthase, the First Enzyme in the MEP Pathway, in Plant Extracts -- Determination of 3-Hydroxy-3-methylglutaryl CoA Reductase Activity in Plants -- Farnesyl Diphosphate Synthase Assay -- Metabolite Profiling of Plastidial Deoxyxylulose-5-Phosphate Pathway Intermediates by Liquid Chromatography and Mass Spectrometry -- Analysis of Carotenoids and Tocopherols in Plant Matrices and Assessment of Their In Vitro Antioxidant Capacity -- Simultaneous Analyses of Oxidized and Reduced Forms of Photosynthetic Quinones by High-Performance Liquid Chromatography -- Determination of Sterol Lipids in Plant Tissues by Gas Chromatography and Q-TOF Mass Spectrometry -- Analysis of Plant Polyisoprenoids -- Analysis of Diterpenes and Triterpenes from Plant Foliage and Roots -- Gas Chromatography Mass-Spectrometry Method for Determination of Biogenic Volatile Organic Compounds Emitted by Plants -- Analysis of Steroidal Alkaloids and Saponins in Solanaceae Plant Extracts

	using UPLC-qTOF Mass Spectrometry -- Isoprenoid and Metabolite Profiling of Plant Trichomes -- Sample Preparation for Single Cell Transcriptomics -- Essential Oil Glands in Citrus Fruit Peel as an Example -- Prenylquinone Profiling in Whole Leaves and Chloroplast Subfractions -- Confocal Laser Scanning Microscopy Detection of Chlorophylls and Carotenoids in Chloroplasts and Chromoplasts of Tomato Fruit -- Heterologous Expression of Triterpene Biosynthetic Genes in Yeast and Subsequent Metabolite Identification Through GC-MS -- High Throughput Testing of Terpenoid Biosynthesis Candidate Genes Using Transient Expression in Nicotiana benthamiana -- Heterologous Stable Expression of Terpenoid Biosynthetic Genes Using the Moss Physcomitrella patens -- Quantification of Plant Resistance to Isoprenoid Biosynthesis Inhibitors -- A Flexible Protocol for Targeted Gene Co-Expression Network Analysis.
Subjects	Isopentenoids--Laboratory manuals. Terpenes--metabolism--Laboratory Manuals. Plants--metabolism--Laboratory Manuals. Terpenes--analysis--Laboratory Manuals. Terpenes--pharmacology--Laboratory Manuals.
Form/Genre	Laboratory Manuals.
Notes	Includes bibliographical references and index.
Series	Methods in molecular biology, 1064-3745; 1153 Springer protocols Methods in molecular biology (Clifton, N.J.); 1153. 1064-3745 Springer protocols (Series) 1949-2448

Plant secondary metabolism engineering: methods and applications

LCCN	2010923085
Type of material	Book
Main title	Plant secondary metabolism engineering: methods and applications / edited by Arthur Germano Fett-Neto.
Published/Created	New York, NY: Springer/Humana Press, c2010.
Description	xii, 339 p.: ill.; 27 cm.

ISBN	9781607617228 (alk. paper) 1607617226 (alk. paper) 9781607617235 (e-ISBN) 1607617234 (e-ISBN)
LC classification	TP248.3 .P53 2010
Related names	Fett-Neto, Arthur Germano, 1967-
Contents	Plant secondary metabolism and challenges in modifying its operation: an overview / Naíla Cannes do Nascimento and Arthur Germano Fett-Neto -- Suppression subtractive hybridization as a tool to identify anthocyanin metabolism-related genes in apple skin / Yusuke Ban and Takaya Moriguchi -- Identification of regulatory protein genes involved in alkaloid biosynthesis using a transient RNAi system / Yasuyuki Yamada ... [et al.] -- Site-directed mutagenesis and saturation mutagenesis for the functional study of transcription factors involved in plant secondary metabolite biosynthesis / Sitakanta Pattanaik ... [et al.] -- Isolation of proteins binding to promoter elements of alkaloid metabolism-related genes using yeast one-hybrid / Débora Vom Endt and Giancarlo Pasquali -- Modulation of carotenoid accumulation in transgenic potato by inducing chromoplast formation with enhanced sink strength / Joyce Van Eck ... [et al.] -- Over-expression of rate-limiting enzymes to improve alkaloid productivity / Tomoya Takemura ... [et al.] -- Microbial expression of alkaloid biosynthetic enzymes for characterization of their properties / Hiromichi Minami, Nobuhiro Ikezawa, and Fumihiko Sato -- Producing a recombinant flavin-containing monooxygenase from Coffea arabica in Escherichia coli for screening of potential natural substrates / Igor Cesarino and Paulo Mazzafera -- Efficient production of active form recombinant cassava hydroxynitrile lyase using Escherichia coli in low-temperature culture / Hisashi Semba ... [et al.] -- Introduction of the early pathway to taxol biosynthesis in yeast by means of biosynthetic gene cluster construction using SOE-PCR and

homologous recombination / Pia Dahm and Stefan Jennewein -- Biocatalytic synthesis of tritium (^3H)-labelled taxa-4(5), 11(12)-diene, the pathway committing precursor of the taxoid diterpenoids / Hans Schmeer and Stefan Jennewein -- USER cloning and USER fusion: the ideal cloning techniques for small and big laboratories / Hussam H. Nour-Eldin, Fernando Geu-Flores, and Barbara A. Halkier -- Enrichment of carotenoids in flaxseed by introducing a bacterial phytoene synthase gene / Masaki Fujisawa and Norihiko Misawa -- Metabolic engineering by plastid transformation as a strategy to modulate isoprenoid yield in plants / Tomohisa Hasunuma, Akihiko Kondo, and Chikahiro Miyake -- Engineering high yields of secondary metabolites in Rubia cell cultures through transformation with rol genes / Victor P. Bulgakov, yuri N. Shkryl, and Galina N. Veremeichik -- Flow cytometric methods to investigate culture heterogeneities for plant metabolic engineering / Vishal Gaurav, Martin E. Kolewe, and Susan C. Roberts -- Phenylpropanoid biosynthesis in leaves and glandular trichomes of basil (Ocimum basilicum L.) / Cícero Deschamps and James E. Simon -- Fusion with fluorescent proteins for subcellular localization of enzymes involved in plant alkaloid biosynthesis / Patrícia Duarte, Johan Memelink, and Mariana Sottomayor -- Immunohistochemical localisation of a putative flavonoid transporter in grape berries / Elisa Petrussa ... [et al.] -- Electrogenic bromosulfalein transport in isolated membrane vesicles: implementation of both animal and plant preparations for the study of flavonoid transporters / Sabina Passamonti ... [et al.]

Subjects

Biochemical engineering--Laboratory manuals.
Plants--Effect of stress on--Research--Laboratory manuals.
Biotransformation (Metabolism)--Research--Laboratory manuals.
Metabolism, Secondary--Research--Laboratory

	manuals.
	Bioengineering--methods--Laboratory Manuals.
	Biotransformation--Laboratory Manuals.
	Plants--metabolism--Laboratory Manuals.
	Research--Laboratory Manuals.
	Biochemical engineering--Laboratory manuals.
	Plants--Effect of stress on--Research--Laboratory manuals.
	Biotransformation (Metabolism)--Research--Laboratory manuals.
	Metabolism, Secondary--Research--Laboratory manuals.
Notes	Includes bibliographical references and index.
Additional formats	Online version: Plant secondary metabolism engineering. New York, NY: Humana Press, c2010 (OCoLC)741941995
Series	Springer protocols Methods in molecular biology, 1064-3745; 643

The future of dynamic structural science

LCCN	2014931397
Type of material	Book
Meeting name	NATO Advanced Study Institute on The Future of Dynamic Structural Science: Links to Energy and Environmental Security and Early Detection of CBRN Agents (2013: Erice, Italy)
Main title	The future of dynamic structural science / edited by Judith A.K. Howard, Department of Chemistry, Durham University, United Kingdom, Hazel A. Sparkes, School of Chemistry, University of Bristol, Bristol, Paul R. Raithby, Department of Chemistry, University of Bath, United Kindom, and Andrei V. Churakov, N.S. Kurnakov Institute of General and Inorganic Chemistry, Russian Academy of Sciences, Moscow, Russia.
Published/Produced	Dordrecht: Springer, 2014.
Description	xvi, 284 pages: illustrations (some color); 24 cm.
Links	Publisher description https://www.loc.gov/catdir/enhancements/fy1617/2014931397-d.html

	Table of contents only https://www.loc.gov/catdir/enhancements/fy1617/2014931397-t.html
ISBN	9789401785525 (hbk) 940178552X (hbk) 9789401785495 940178549X
LC classification	QD901 .N373 2013
Related names	Howard, J. A. K., editor. Sparkes, Hazel A., editor. Raithby, P. R. (Paul R.), editor. Churakov, Andrei V., editor.
Summary	This work focuses on complementary crystallographic and spectroscopic areas of dynamic structural science, from papers presented at the 46th NATO sponsored course in Erice, Sicily 2013. These papers cover a range of material from background concepts to more advanced material and represent a fully inter-disciplinary collection of the latest ideas and results within the field. They will appeal to practising or novice crystallographers, both chemical and biological, who wish to learn more about modern spectroscopic methods and convergent advances and hence vice versa for experimental and computational spectroscopists. The chapters refer to the latest techniques, software and results and each chapter is fully referenced. The volume provides an excellent starting point for new comers in the emerging, multi-disciplinary area of time resolved science.-- Source other than the Library of Congress.
Contents	Single Crystal and Powder Methods for Structure Determination of Metastable Species -- Raman Crystallography, the Missing Link between Biochemical Reactions and Crystallography -- Structure and Dynamics from Time Resolved Absorption and Raman Spectroscopy -- Time and Space-Resolved Spectroscopy -- Dynamic X-Ray and Neutron Scattering: From Materials Synthesis and In-Situ Studies to Biology at High Pressure -- Dynamics of Mechanochemical Processes -- Measuring and

Understanding Ultrafast Phenomena Using X-Rays -- Single-Crystal to Single-Crystal Solid-State Photochemistry -- Femtoseconds to Hours Structural Dynamics Investigations: What do the Different Time Scales tell us in Chemistry? -- Structure and Dynamics of Light-Excited States -- Direct Observation of Various Reaction Pathways in Crystalline State Photoreactions -- Time Resolved XAS Spectroscopy Probing Dynamic Species in Homogeneous Catalysis -- Towards faster Methods Providing more Information -- Dynamical Aspects of Biomacromolecular Multi-Resolution Modelling Using the Ultra Scan Solution Modeler (US-SOMO) Suite -- Linking Diffraction, XAFS and Spectroscopic Studies on Short Lived Species -- Structure Analyses of Unstable Reaction Intermediates Using the Technique of Acid-Base Complex or Polymorphic Crystal Formation -- Molecular Mechanisms of Light-Harvesting and Photo-Protection by Carotenoids Explaining Configurational Selections by Antenna and Reaction Centre Complexes -- Time-Resolved Macromolecular Crystallography in Practice at Bio CARS, Advanced Photon Source: from Data Collection to Structures of Intermediates -- Combining Single Crystal UV/Vis Spectroscopy and Diffraction to Structurally Characterise Intermediates and Monitor Radiation Damage -- Molecular Dynamics Probed by Short X-Ray Pulses from a Synchrotron.

Subjects Crystallography--Congresses.
Crystals--Spectra--Congresses.
Crystallography.
Crystals--Spectra.

Form/Genre Conference proceedings.

Notes "Proceedings of the NATO Advanced Study Institute on The Future of Dynamic Structural Science: Links to Energy and Environmental Security and Early Detection of CBRN Agents, Erice, Italy, 30 May - 8 June, 2013."
NATO Science for Peace and Security Series A:

Series	Chemistry and Biology, 1874-6489 NATO science for peace and security series. Series A, Chemistry and biology. 1874-6489

Vegetables, whole grains, and their derivatives in cancer prevention

LCCN	2010936635
Type of material	Book
Main title	Vegetables, whole grains, and their derivatives in cancer prevention / Marja Mutanen, Anne-Maria Pajari, editors.
Published/Created	Dordrecht; New York: Springer, c2011.
Description	xvii, 250 p.: ill.; 25 cm.
ISBN	9789048197996 (alk. paper) 9048197996 (alk. paper)
LC classification	RC268.45 .V44 2011
Related names	Mutanen, Marja. Pajari, Anne-Maria.
Contents	Diet and cancer, how to prevent or cure tumors with the help of food, beverages, and their derivatives -- Cruciferous vegetables-and biological activity of isothiocyanates and indoles / Richard Mithen, Charlotte Armah, and Maria Traka -- Green leafy vegetables in cancer prevention / Marja Mutanen, Mikael Niku, and Seija Oikarinen -- The role of tomato lycopene in cancer prevention / Joseph Levy ... [et al.] -- [beta]-carotene and other carotenoids in cancer prevention / Yan Wang and Xiang-Dong Wang -- The role of alliums and their sulfur and selenium constituents in cancer prevention / Karam El-Bayoumy ... [et al.] -- Molecular mechanisms of chemoprevention with capsaicinoids from chili peppers / Young-Joon Surh and Joydeb Kumar Kundu -- Influence of dietary soy isoflavones genistein and daidzein on genotoxicity and mammary carcinogenicity in rats exposed to the model carcinogen 7,12-dimethylbenz[a]anthracene (DMBA) / Anane Aidoo and Mugimane G. Manjanatha -- The potential roles of seeds and seed bioactives on the prevention and treatment of breast and prostate cancer

/ Krista A. Power and Lilian U. Thompson -- Nuts as part of a whole diet approach to cancer prevention / Paul A. Davis -- Whole grains and their constituents in the prevention of colon cancer / Anne-Maria Pajari.

Subjects Cancer--Nutritional aspects.
Cancer--Prevention.
Neoplasms--diet therapy.
Neoplasms--prevention & control.
Cereals.
Diet Therapy.
Vegetables.

Notes Includes bibliographical references and index.

Series Diet and cancer; 2

RELATED NOVA PUBLICATIONS

CAROTENOIDS: FOOD SOURCES, PRODUCTION AND HEALTH BENEFITS

Editors: Masayoshi Yamaguchi
Department of Hematology and Medical Oncology,
Emory University School of Medicine, Atlanta, GA, US

ISBN: 978-1-62808-622-5 Publication Date: 2013

Carotenoids are the most widespread pigments in nature. One or more carotenoids in combination give rise to colors ranging from yellow to red in birds, fishes, crustaceans, microorganisms, fruits and plants, including the dark green ones. There are over 600 known carotenoids and they are divided into two classes: xanthophylls, which contain oxygen, and carotenes, which are purely hydrocarbons and contain no oxygen. Carotenoids have many health benefits including antioxidant properties, free-radical scavengers, decreasing the risk of cardiovascular disease, anti-inflammatory properties, osteoporosis prevention and other diseases. The 15 chapters in this book have been written to outline recent topical research.

Chapter 1 - Carotenoids as Bioactive Compounds
Authors / Editors: (Aline Inácio Alves, Afonso Mota Ramos, Paulo César Stringheta and Ellen Silva Lago Vanzela, Universidade Federal de Viçosa –

UFV, Peter Henry Rolfs, s/n, Campus Universitário, Viçosa, Minas Gerais, Brazil, and others)

Chapter 2 - Food Sources: Production and Health Benefits of Carotenoids

Authors / Editors: (Lucia Maria Jaeger de Carvalho, Lara de Azevedo Sarmet Moreira Smiderle, Ediane Maria Gomes Ribeiro, Gisela Dellamora Ortiz, Patrícia Barros Gomes and José Luiz Viana de Carvalho, Federal University of Rio de Janeiro, Faculty of Pharmacy, Ilha do Fundão, Rio de Janeiro, Brazil, and others)

Chapter 3 - Carotenoids with κ-End Group

Authors / Editors: (Enrique Murillo, Veronika Nagy, Attila Agócs and József Deli, University of Panamá, Biochemistry and Nutrition Laboratory, Panama, and others)

Chapter 4 - Development of a Method to Induce ROS Resistant High-Yielding Mutant Lines of Sugar Cane, *Saccharum officinarum* cv NiF8 and NiTn18

Authors / Editors: (Kohji Hasunuma, Yusuke Yoshida, Md Emdadul Haque, Yosuke Fukamatsu, Yoshifumi Terajima and Makoto Matsuoka, Kihara Institute for Biological Research, Yokohama City University, Kanagawa, Japan, and others)

Chapter 5 - Molecular Base for Carotenoids Antioxidant Activity in Model and Biological Systems: The Health-Related Effects

Authors / Editors: (Dragan Cvetkovic, Leszek Fiedor, Joanna Fiedor, Anna Wisniewska-Becker and Dejan Markovic, Faculty of Technology, University of Nish, Leskovac, Serbia, and others)

Chapter 6 - Carotenoids in Herbal Medicines

Authors / Editors: (Mamta Kshipra Misra, Kshipra Misra, Satinder Kaur Brar and Mausam Verma, Defence Institute of Physiology and Allied Sciences, Lucknow Road, Timarpur, Delhi, India, and others)

Chapter 7 - Microalgae: A Valuable Source of Natural Carotenoids with Potential Health Benefits

Authors / Editors: (Faruq Ahmed, Kent Fanning, Holger Schuhmann, Michael Netzel and Peer Schenk, School of Agriculture and Food Science, The University of Queensland, St Lucia, QLD, Australia, and others)

Chapter 8 - Sodium Taurocholate Optimum Amount of Blood Parrots on Astaxanthin Availability

Authors / Editors: (Xidong Mu, Huiyun Yang, Yinchang Hu and Jianren Luo, Pearl River Fisheries Research Institute, Chinese Academy of Fishery Sciences, Key Laboratory of Tropical & Subtropical Fishery Resource Application & Cultivation, Ministry of Agriculture, Guangzhou, China)

Chapter 9 - Carotenoid-Based Ornaments as Signals of Health Status in Birds: Evidences from Two Galliform Species, the Red-Legged Partridge (*Alectoris rufa*) and the Red Grouse (*Lagopus lagopus scoticus*)

Authors / Editors: (Lorenzo Pérez-Rodríguez, Jesús Martínez-Padilla and François Mougeot, CIBIO, Centro de Investigação em Biodiversidade e Recursos Genéticos, Campus Agrário de Vairão, Vairão, Portugal and others)

Chapter 10 - Dietary Carotenoid Pigments and Human Health Benefits

Authors / Editors: (Hasna El Gharras, Laboratoire de Chimie Organique et Analytique. Unité de Chimie Agroalimentaire, Université Sultan Moulay Slimane, Faculté des Sciences et Techniques, Béni-Mellal, Morocco)

Chapter 11 - Health Benefits of Carotenoids for Human Skin

Authors / Editors: (Maxim E. Darvin and Juergen Lademann, Charité - Universitätsmedizin Berlin, Department of Dermatology, Venerology and Allergology, Center of Experimental and Applied Cutaneous Physiology (CCP), Berlin, Germany)

Chapter 12 - Nanoparticles of Chitin Nanofibril-Hyaluronan Block Polymer Entrapping Lutein as UVA Protective Compound

Authors / Editors: (P. Morganti, H.D. Chen, X.H. Gao, P. Del Ciotto, F. Carezzi and G. Morganti, Dermatology Depart, 2nd University of Naples, Italy, and others)

Chapter 13 - Bixin and Norbixin: Chemistry, Production and Health Benefits

Authors / Editors: (Miguel Roehrs and Rafael Roehrs, Post-graduate Program of Pharmacology, Center of Healthy Sciences, Santa Maria, Brazil, Clinical Laboratory, University Hospital of Santa Maria, Federal University of Santa Maria, Santa Maria, Brazil, and others)

Chapter 14 - Biology of Carotenoids and their Potential Cardiovascular Health Benefits

Authors / Editors: (Assunta Pandolfi, Department of Experimental and Clinical Sciences, "G. d'Annunzio" University, Italy and others)

Chapter 15 - Effects of Carotenoids on Mammalian DNA Polymerase Inhibition and Anti-Inflammatory Activity

Authors / Editors: (Yoshiyuki Mizushina, Isoko Kuriyama, Toshifumi Takeuchi, Fumio Sugawara and Hiromi Yoshida, Laboratory of Food & Nutritional Sciences, Faculty of Nutrition, Kobe Gakuin University, Nishi-ku, Kobe, Hyogo, Japan, and others)

Chapter 16 - Dietary β-Cryptoxanthin Stimulates Osteogenesis: Role in Prevention and Treatment of Osteoporosis

Authors / Editors: (Masayoshi Yamaguchi, Department of Hematology and Medical Oncology, Emory University School of Medicine, Atlanta, GA, USA)

MICROBIAL CAROTENOIDS: PROPERTIES, PHYSICOCHEMICAL FACTORS FOR FERMENTATION, BIOSYNTHESIS AND APPLICATIONS*

***Krupa Patel*[1], *Dweipayan Goswami*[1], *Pinakin Dhandhukia*[2] and *Janki N. Thakker*[1,†]**

[1]Department of Biotechnology, P.D. Patel Institute of Applied Sciences, Charotar University of Science and Technology, CHARUSAT Campus, Changa, Anand (Gujarat), India

[2]Ashok and Rita Patel Institute of Integrated Study and Research in Biotechnology and Allied Sciences, ADIT Campus, New Vidyangar, Anand (Gujarat), India

Natural products, due to their diverse structures and applications, have more importance in pharmaceutical and food industries compared to synthetic products. One such product is pigments of natural origin like chlorophyll, melanins, carotenoids, etc. Among various natural sources, microbial carotenoids are available in different forms having application in food, nutraceutical and pharmaceutical industries. Carotenoids are structurally categorized into two classes: carotenes (e.g., lycopene, α-carotene, and β-carotene), which are exclusively hydrocarbons, and xanthophylls (e.g., lutein, α-cryptoxanthin and β-cryptoxanthin, zeaxanthin, canthaxanthin and astaxanthin), which are oxygenated. Depending on the number of double bond formation with phytoene structure different type of carotenoids are derived and shows a signature absorbance pattern in the 300–600 nm range, which gives them typical colors like red, yellow, orange, etc. More than 700 different types of carotenoids are known, derived using two different pathways, mevalonic acid pathway and 2-C-methyl-D-erythritol 4-phosphate/ 1-deoxy-D-xylulose 5-phosphate pathway (MEP/DOXP pathway). Carotenoid desaturase,

---

* The full version of this chapter can be found in *Microbes in Action*, edited by Neelam Garg and Abhinav Aeron, published by Nova Science Publishers, Inc, New York, 2016.

† Corresponding Author: Dr. Janki N. Thakker, Department of Biotechnology, P.D. Patel Institute of Applied Sciences, Charotar University of Science and Technology, CHARUSAT Campus, Changa-388421, Anand (Gujarat), India, Phone: +91-2697-247500/248133*2194, Fax: +91-2697-247100, E-mail: jankithakker.bt@ecchanga.ac.in.

carotenoid cyclase and carotenoid oxygenase are three major enzymes that lead to the formation of different carotenoid molecules. The interest in the production of natural carotenoids by microbial fermentation has increased and they are considered biotechnologically high-value compounds with an annual market estimated to have exceeded one billion US dollars till date. By changing physicochemical factors like medium components, *pH* of media, temperature, aeration, presence of inorganic salts and an organic carbon source of the medium, the type and amount of carotenoid differs in a microorganism. Carotenogenic microbes such as *Dunaliella salina*, *Xanthophyllomyces dendrorhous*, *Haematococcu spluvialis*, and *Blakeslea trispora* have been investigated for large-scale production because of its cost effectiveness. Scientific interest in dietary carotenoids has increased in recent years because of their beneficial effects on human health, such as lowering the risk of cancer and enhancement of immune system function, preventing the cell from damage which is ascribed by their antioxidant potential. Carotenoids play a major role in quenching singlet oxygen radicals and removing molecular oxygen from the biological system without producing any oxidizing products. Present chapter focuses on the sources of microbial carotenoids, types of carotenoids, factors affecting the carotenoid production, market status of microbial carotenoids and their applications.

CAROTENOIDS BIOSYNTHESIS IN *CORYNEBACTERIUM GLUTAMICUM*[*]

Miriam Martínez-Castro, Esther Bahíllo, Sonia Martínez-Cámara and José-Luis Barredo[†]
Gadea Biopharma, Parque Tecnológico de León, León, Spain

Carotenoids are a family of yellow to orange-red terpenoid pigments synthesized by photosynthetic organisms and by many bacteria and fungi.

[*] The full version of this chapter can be found in *New Trends in Corynebacterium glutamicum: Beyond the Amino Acids*, edited by Carlos Barreiro, published by Nova Science Publishers, Inc, New York, 2015.

[†] Corresponding Author Email: joseluis.barredo@gadea.com.

They are involved in diverse functions such as photo-protection, light harvesting and as membrane stabilizers. They show beneficial health effects, protecting against oxidative damage, and being responsible of the colours associated with many plants and animals. Animals must obtain the carotenoids through their diet, having some of them important functions as precursors of vitamin A and different hormones. Carotenoids are commercially used as food colorants, animal feed supplements, and cosmetics as well as in the nutraceutical and pharmaceutical industries. Only a few of the hundreds of identified carotenoids are industrially produced, being β-carotene the most prominent. *Corynebacterium glutamicum* is a known producer of decaprenoxanthin, a glycosylated C_{50} yellow pigment. After elucidation of the decaprenoxanthin biosynthetic pathway, metabolic engineering was used to construct a lycopene producing strain of *C. glutamicum* as a platform for the production of different C_{50} and C_{40} carotenoids. The productivities of lycopene, β-carotene, zeaxanthin, C.p.450, sarcinaxanthin and decaprenoxanthin by recombinant strains of *C. glutamicum* are in the range of milligram per gram of dry weight.

Biosynthesis, Analysis and Antioxidant Properties of Tocols and Carotenoids from Corn Oil*

Vasile Robert Gradinaru[1,†]
and Luiza Madalina Gradinaru[2]
[1]Department of Chemistry, "Alexandru Ioan Cuza" University, Iasi, Romania
[2]"Petru Poni" Institute of Macromolecular Chemistry, Iasi, Romania

Corn oil is an edible oil extracted from the maize germ and has multiple applications. This chapter focuses on biosynthesis, analysis and antitoxidant

* The full version of this chapter can be found in *Corn and Coconut Oil: Antioxidant Properties, Uses and Health Benefits*, edited by Constantin Apetrei, published by Nova Science Publishers, Inc, New York, 2015.

† Corresponding Author E-mail: robert.gradinaru@uaic.ro.

activity of two classes of compounds, tocols and carotenoids, which are present in this vegetal oil. The demand to obtain corn oil with high levels of antioxidants should be considered. Tremendous work has been carried out in order to increase the level of these antioxidants by switching or modifying biochemical pathways. However, new approaches should be taken into consideration in order to increase their concentration in corn oil. A whole range of analysis or estimation methods of antioxidant activy are presented herein. The data suggest that tocopherols, as well as carotenoids, from corn oil are important antioxidant molecules. Moreover, development of more specific detection assays to distinguish their individual contribution to the total antioxidant activity should be taken into account.

MICROALGAE AS SOURCE OF HIGH ADDED-VALUE COMPOUNDS: CAROTENOIDS*

León Sánchez[1] and Marcia Morales[2]

[1]Doctorado en Biotecnología, Universidad Autónoma Metropolitana-Iztapalapa, México, DF, Mexico

[2]Departamento de Procesos y Tecnología, Universidad Autónoma Metropolitana-Cuajimalpa, colonia Santa Fe Cuajimalpa, México, DF, Mexico

Microalgae can be used as cell factories (biofactories) for the industrial production of carotenoids. Carotenoids are high-value chemicals with health benefits. An economically feasible production of carotenoids with microalgae is possible because microalgae produce these compounds directly from the solar energy at high photosynthetic efficiencies. In addition, microalgal production systems have high volumetric and areal productivities. Research contribution in biosynthesis, metabolic regulation, and metabolic engineering of carotenoids will support the future exploration of novel carotenoid production strategies. However, it is necessary to improve culture methods and

* The full version of this chapter can be found in *Microalgae and Other Phototrophic Bacteria: Culture, Processing, Recovery and New Products*, edited by Luis G. Torres Bustillos, published by Nova Science Publishers, Inc, New York, 2015.

downstream processing because they represent the major challenge in the massive production due to the high cost and energy requirement.

ADVANCES IN STUDY OF CAROTENOIDS IN CITRUS FRUIT*

Xiangyu Li[1], Juan Li[2] and Jiezhong Chen[1,†]
[1] College of Horticulture, South China Agricultural University, Guangzhou, China
[2] Department of Horticulture, Zhongkai University of Agriculture and Engineering, Guangzhou, China

Carotenoids, which are a class of important natural pigments, endow plants with yellow, orange and red color, and play crucial functions in photosynthesis and synthesis of abscisic acid. In addition, carotenoids are closely related to human health. Recent studies suggest that carotenoids are not only the precursor of vitamin A, but also play important roles in antioxidant capacity, human immunity improvement and cancer prevention. Citrus is rich in bioactive compounds and has been an excellent source of carotenoids for humans and other animals. So, putting effort into the research and development of citrus carotenoids is worthwhile. In this article we reviewed the composition, biosynthesis and regulation of carotenoids in citrus fruit, and the various biological functions such as the antioxidant property, light protective effects and anticancer effect.

---

* The full version of this chapter can be found in *Citrus: Molecular Phylogeny, Antioxidant Properties and Medicinal Uses*, edited by Khizar Hayat, published by Nova Science Publishers, Inc, New York, 2014.

† Corresponding Author: E-mail: cjzlxb@scau.edu.cn.

Carotenoids and Cardiovascular Disease*

Graziano Riccioni†
Human and Clinical Nutrition Unit, Department of Biomedical Science, Via Dei Vestini, University G. D'Annunzio, Chieti-Pescara, Italy.
Cardiology Unit, San Camillo De Lellis Hospital, Manfredonia, FG, Italy.

Carotenoids are a class of natural fat-soluble pigments found principally in plants with potential antioxidant biological properties because of their chemical structure and interaction with biological membranes.

Numerous epidemiologic studies supported the hypothesis that antioxidants could be used as an inexpensive means of both primary and secondary cardiovascular disease (CVD) prevention. In fact, the oxidation of low-density lipoproteins (LDL) in the vessels plays a key role in the development of atherosclerotic lesions and CVD.

The resistance of LDL to oxidation is increased by antioxidant supplementation: consequently, high intake of antioxidants leads to a decreased risk of coronary heart disease (CHD). Further, properties of carotenoids leading to reduction of cardiovascular risk are represented by lowering of blood pressure, reduction of proinflammatory cytokines and markers of inflammation (such as C-reactive protein), improvement of insulin sensitivity in muscle, liver and adipose tissues.

In addition recently nutrigenomics studies have focused on the exceptional ability of carotenoids in modulating the expression of specific genes involved in cell metabolism. The aim of this chapter is to point out the attention to the effects of many carotenoids in the prevention of CVD.

---

* The full version of this chapter can be found in *Nutraceuticals and Functional Foods: Natural Remedy*, edited by Satinder Kaur Brar, Surinder Kaur and Gurpreet Singh Dhillon, published by Nova Science Publishers, Inc, New York, 2013.

† Corresponding Author E-mail: griccioni@hotmail.com.

THE HEALTH EFFECTS ON CAROTENOIDS OF KIWIFRUITS (*ACTINIDIA SPP.*) BASED ON THEIR EVIDENCES*

***Noboru Motohashi*†**

Meiji Pharmaceutical University, Kiyose-shi, Tokyo, Japan

Kiwifruits (*Actinidia spp.*) could be divided into both tender and hardy kiwifruits. Therefore, their kiwifruits adapted to the natural features and climate of the area have been begun to cultivate worldwide, especially, in New Zealand, USA, Korea, China, Japan and others.

It has been found that the consumption of daily kiwifruits could reduce their platelet aggregation and plasma lipids in healthy human volunteers, and especially the kiwifruit carotenoids could reveal two properties such as their provitamin A activity and antioxidant capacity for their excess and harmful reactive oxygen species (ROS) in human body and a yellow plant pigment lutein might be useful for the improvement on macular degeneration of a degeneration of the macular pigment) in human eyes happened by aging. Especially, the antioxidative kiwifruit carotenoids with mainly yellow-orange or red colors such as α-carotene (1), β-carotene (2), lutein (6) and β-cryptoxanthin (5) might be beneficial to their prevention and treatment of the age-related diseases such as macular degeneration, hypertension, heart failure and diabetes by the scavenging activity of reactive oxygen species (ROS).

Based on these evidences of their kiwifruit carotenoids, the purpose of this review is to describe their source and health effects on mainly the kiwifruit carotenoids such as xanthophylls and carotenoids.

* The full version of this chapter can be found in *Occurrences, Structure, Biosynthesis, and Health Benefits Based on Their Evidences of Medicinal Phytochemicals in Vegetables and Fruits. Volume 1*, edited by Noboru Motohashi, published by Nova Science Publishers, Inc, New York, 2013.

† Corresponding Author Email: noborumotohashi@jcom.home.ne.jp.

Carotenoids and Adiposity[*]

J. Atilio Canas[†]
Mayo Medical School, Department of Pediatric Endocrinology, Diabetes and Metabolism, Nemours Children's Clinic, Jacksonville, FL, US

In recent years, the world has seen an alarming increase in metabolic diseases including obesity, insulin resistance, diabetes, fatty liver disease, and atherosclerosis. Recent studies have clearly identified adipose tissue as a critical site for whole body metabolic regulation via carotenoid metabolism and storage.

A growing body of evidence supports the concept that the bioavailability of dietary carotenoids and their metabolic products (retinoids) not only provide protection against oxidative stress but also act as nuclear regulatory factors interlinking adipocytes, with vitamin A metabolism. These actions include growth and proliferation, regulation of fuel metabolism, adipokine production, and constitute an important component of the endocrine effects of this organ, on systemic carbohydrate and lipid homeostasis.

Several large epidemiological studies have shown a correlation between lower plasma carotenoid levels and increased risk of obesity, metabolic syndrome (MetS), type 2 diabetes (T2DM) and cardiovascular disease (CVD). Food based interventional studies suggest that specifically increased consumption of green leafy vegetables, which are important dietary sources of carotenoids, have been associated with reduced risk for T2DM and CVD.

In contrast, the interpretation of adult carotenoid supplementation trials with supra-physiological doses of single or a few combined vitamins, have been mixed for disease prevention, and may even show detrimental effects.

---

[*] The full version of this chapter can be found in *Beta-Carotene: Functions, Health Benefits and Adverse Effects*, edited by Maxime Lefevre, published by Nova Science Publishers, Inc, New York, 2012.

[†] Corresponding Author Email: jcanas@nemours.org.

Consequently, there is a critical need to evaluate the effects of whole food or whole food supplements in the prevention of obesity and its related metabolic dysregulation. In this Chapter, the evidence for a role of carotenoids and its metabolites in adipocyte biology will be evaluated, and the rational for establishing recommended daily intakes and desirable serum and tissue levels, through well designed epidemiological studies, will be proposed.

INDEX

D

E

F

G

H

I

K

L

M

N

O

P

Q

R

S